Praise for *How to Get the Right Diagnosis*

"If you, or one of your loved ones, has a complex, chronic illness, you need to read this book. You are not alone if you fear your medical problems are misunderstood. This book, written by an analyst of the highest caliber, Randolph Pherson, teaches you how to take charge of your own healthcare in an organized, structured way. As a physician, I am happy to give my strong endorsement to Mr. Pherson's advice that you need a doctor who will spend time with you and will look for root causes of symptoms. Follow Pherson's advice: if both the doctor and the patient ask a lot of questions to get a complete picture, then, chances are, you will discover the true diagnosis."

—Dr. Jeanne Shiffman, Well Being–Being Well, Integrative and Family Medicine

"Mr. Pherson deftly applies his decades of experience practicing, developing, and teaching the art of intelligence to the life and death issue of accurate medical diagnoses. He goes beyond the message that patients must advocate for their health to provide a practical roadmap for partnering with medical professionals to solve non-obvious medical challenges. His book is a must read for medical professionals to ensure they are challenging their assumptions and considering alternative scenarios. But more importantly, it is a must read for anyone facing a seemingly undiagnosable, but potentially life-threatening medical issue."

—Fran Moore, former Director of Intelligence, Central Intelligence Agency

"Doctors want to be thought of as all-knowing, but they cannot be all-knowing, since the screening testing they prescribe often leaves a large level of doubt. Physicians should offer more information to the patient specific to that level of doubt, but often, they do not take the time to explain "false normals" that can occur at rates as high as 20 percent. Randy's story is a great example of why all of us, as patients, need to demand full disclosure on all medical testing and insist on clear answers about tests that are not perfect."

—**Doug Boyink**, MD, Fellow, American College of
Emergency Physicians

"Randolph Pherson's distinguished career as a senior intelligence officer and author has had a significant impact internationally on the professionalisation of analysts working in national security and law enforcement. This time, he applies, in a novel and personal way, the critical thinking and tradecraft knowledge he has gained in the intelligence world to improving the diagnostic skills of the medical profession. The book is a must read for an increasingly time-starved and hyper-specialised medical profession and a useful resource for patients seeking better health advocacy with their doctors."

—**Patrick F. Walsh**, Associate Professor, Charles Sturt
University, Australia

HOW TO GET

THE RIGHT

DIAGNOSIS

Also by Randolph H. Pherson

Structured Analytic Techniques for Intelligence Analysis, 3rd ed., Randolph H. Pherson and Richards J. Heuer, Jr., Washington DC, CQ Press/SAGE Publications, 2021.

Critical Thinking for Strategic Intelligence, 2nd ed., Katherine Hibbs Pherson and Randolph H. Pherson. Washington, DC: CQ Press/SAGE Publications, 2017.

Cases in Intelligence Analysis: Structured Analytic Techniques in Action, 2nd ed., Sarah Miller Beebe and Randolph H. Pherson. Washington, DC: CQ Press/SAGE Publications, 2015.

Handbook of Analytic Tools and Techniques, 5th ed., Randolph H. Pherson. Tysons, VA: Pherson Associates, 2019.

Analyst's Guide to Indicators, Randolph H. Pherson and John Pyrik. Tysons, VA: Pherson Associates, 2018.

Analytic Briefing Guide, Randolph H. Pherson, Walter Voskian, and Roy A. Sullivan, Jr. Reston, VA: Pherson Associates, 2018.

Analytic Production Guide, Walter Voskian and Randolph H. Pherson. Reston, VA: Pherson Associates, 2016.

Analytic Writing Guide, Louis Kaiser and Randolph H. Pherson. Reston, VA: Pherson Associates, 2014.

Intelligence Communication in the Digital Era: Transforming Security, Defence and Business, Rubén Arcos and Randolph H. Pherson, editors. London: Palgrave Macmillan, 2015.

Rethinking Intelligence: Richards J. Heuer, Jr.'s Life of Public Service, Richards J. Heuer Jr., Randolph H. Pherson, editor. Tysons, VA: Pherson Associates, 2018.

To order any of these publications, go to:

shop.globalytica.com/collections/publications

HOW TO GET THE RIGHT DIAGNOSIS

16 Tips for Navigating the Medical System

Randolph H. Pherson

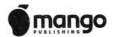

Mango Publishing

CORAL GABLES

Mango Publishing Group
2850 Douglas Road, 2nd Floor
Coral Gables, FL 33134 USA
info@mango.bz

For special orders, quantity sales, course adoptions and corporate sales, please email the publisher at sales@mango. bz. For trade and wholesale sales, please contact Ingram Publisher Services at customer.service@ingramcontent.com or +1.800.509.4887.

How to Get the Right Diagnosis: 16 Tips for Navigating the Medical System

Library of Congress Cataloging
ISBN: (p) 978-1-64250-176-6 (e) 978-1-64250-177-3

BISAC: MED074000, MEDICAL / Physician & Patient

LCCN: 2019948634

Printed in the United States of America

To those in the "5 percent club" who died not knowing they were members.

Table of Contents

Foreword by Sandy Ibrahim, MD

In medical school, one of the questions I was taught to ask a distressed patient was, "Do you have a sense of impending doom?" What a silly thing to say, I thought. Who even talks like that? I have labs and tests that will answer that question better. ECGs, for example, can tell me much more than a patient could ever relate. I practice in the nation's capital, and it is easy to send a patient down the street for fancy imaging, nuclear tests, or even the "million-dollar workup," paid for by his insurance.

That being the case, why would I ask such a ridiculous question? Why would I put my diagnosis at the mercy of a patient's answer to this outdated textbook question? Who would know best? The patient or a trained physician?

By the time Randy Pherson walked into my office, I had run out of diagnostic testing options that would explain his ever-persistent shortness of breath. We had spent five years exhausting the pathways of modern medicine. I had sent him to multiple specialists who ordered scores of diagnostic tests and prescribed multiple treatments. Unfortunately, every path led to a dead end. So, I fell back to asking that old school question: "Does Randy exhibit a strange sense of impending doom?"

Asking that question likely saved his life that day. Randy was tired, frustrated, and at the end of his rope. His face had that look of impending doom, which I had learned about but never encountered until that day. I told him to drive immediately to an emergency room. He protested, saying he would go right after two appointments that afternoon. I countered in no uncertain terms: "You must pick a hospital and drive there now. Non-negotiable."

Over the course of my career, I learned that no matter what diagnostic tools doctors have at their fingertips, the most important route to effective treatment is old-fashioned face-to-face communication, eye contact, and spending quality time with your patients. Specialists should treat the patient, not just order and process test results.

Randy and I are grateful that one emergency room doctor listened to him—although it took a lot of prodding. Physicians need to talk—and better yet, listen—to the patient. They should ask open-ended questions, despite time constraints. They should encourage patients to tell their story instead of just responding to their questions. Doctors need to review patients' data, not just focus on their test results. They should pick up the phone and converse with specialists. Above all, doctors need to learn how to collaborate, brainstorm, and personally engage. It could prove the difference between life and death for those "tough" cases that comprise Randy's "5 percent."

Patients have much to learn from Randy's story as well. They should take responsibility for their own bodies and embrace the concept of preventative medicine. Patients should get annual exams so their doctor has a baseline for tracking their health. The average primary care provider has over three thousand patients under his or her care, and it is hard to remember everyone. If you see your doctor annually to get that wellness exam, we will remember you when you return and need our help. The wellness visit is our opportunity to engage and learn about you and your lifestyle when you are well. When you come in with a medical problem—as in Randy's case, with severe shortness of breath—then your doctor can better gauge the severity of your condition.

With Randy, the objective findings did not match the subjective complaints, but I knew him and saw him often for well visits and sick visits. That knowledge buttressed my confidence in my belief that something was very, very wrong. Doomsday wrong.

As a primary care provider, I am forever humbled by the limitations of modern medicine and amazed at the human body's ability to adapt. What follows is Randy's story of persistence, physical adaptation, and lessons learned in his (our) journey through the pitfalls of modern medicine. I am grateful he is here to share his story with all of you.

Sandy Ibrahim, MD
Medical Director, Inova VIP360
Fairfax, Virginia
January 31, 2019

Foreword by John Gannon

Randy Pherson and I were fellow analysts and friends over long careers at the CIA. We worked together closely in the final years of our careers on the National Intelligence Council where I served as chairman for four years. Randy was an outstanding National Intelligence Officer (NIO) for Latin America during a turbulent time in the region. He was widely respected for his energetic advancement of analytic tradecraft in the information age and for his aggressive outreach to outside sources of expertise in the early post-Cold War period—passions that he brought to improving the quality of analytic tradecraft after retiring from the CIA.

In his thought-provoking book, *How to Get the Right Diagnosis,* Randy notes that intelligence analysts and medical personnel face similar challenges in collecting reliable data to reduce uncertainty and sharpen diagnoses. He reveals how the methodologies and practices he employed so successfully in the US Intelligence Community can also help fill data gaps and contribute to a more complete and accurate medical diagnosis. In this book, he methodically lays out practical prescriptions for prevention, response, and recovery.

Both of us were avid runners who prided ourselves on staying in shape to meet the demands of our often-stressful work. Yet we both surprised ourselves and shocked our families and friends by having life-threatening medical conditions. Randy's story, typical of an intensely curious analyst with a healthy bent toward skepticism, is about his forceful challenge to medical experts. The experts believed they had a better grasp of available data on his evolving diagnosis than he did—and turned out to be wrong.

My story parallels Randy's in many ways. It begins with my own failure to question flawed assumptions about the correlation between apparent good health and immunity from heart disease. I was an in-shape nonsmoker, a sensible eater with no significant family history of diabetes or heart disease. With eight marathons under my belt, I continued to jog regularly, swim every day, and play tennis twice a week. I thought I was in top condition until I almost died from a heart attack after a stressful day in the rugged hills of western Croatia. Unlike Randy who took charge of his medical care, I blame myself for not working with a primary care physician to monitor a growing blood pressure problem related to cholesterol. The alarming data would have been discovered had I sought it—what we sometimes refer to as an "unknown known."

The author's recommendations flow from the basic admonition to take charge, be a proactive participant in your diagnosis and treatment, listen attentively to your own body, ask your doctors every hard question that comes to mind, express doubts when you have them, take notes to help organize and prioritize your issues and concerns, collect your own data to fill inevitable gaps, and keep a data-rich account of your medical history. Above all, never settle on being a passive consumer of your medical data or a silent observer of medical systems and practices. You should interact constantly and vigorously with your doctors and other medical personnel.

In closing, I would like to offer two personal observations related to emotions that go beyond the usual medical discussion of innovative medical procedures and pathbreaking drug therapies. Lots of empirical evidence speaks to the wider relevance of my issues to health. The first is the role of stress in elevating the chances of a heart attack and slowing recovery. This is not that complicated. I know from personal experience that we simply can and should learn to reduce the stress in our lives as an investment in good health. Second is the impact of human relationships.

From the moment I arrived at a Croatian ICU, I believed I could and would get better. I was kept grounded with high morale by the constant reassuring presence of my wife, Mary Ellen, and by the loving support of our children, grandchildren, and close friends. These folks were a powerful driver in my survival and recovery. I'm not sending a Hallmark card here. I'm providing hard data you can take to the bank. Investment in people pays rich dividends!

The good news for Randy and me is that the excellent medical procedures and continuing care we received in the same Northern Virginia hospital, our healthy diets, our regular physical exercise, and our robust network of close family and friends have boosted our resilience and speeded our recovery, turning a brush with death into a wake-up call—a second chance for a long, active life with the people we love. We are still here to tell our stories. We are lucky guys, and we know it!

Randy Pherson made himself a proactive participant in the diagnosis and treatment of his condition and, ultimately, in saving his own life. This gripping story and the sound advice he offers are certain to help others take charge of their health care. We all should take his good advice to heart!

John Gannon
Former Chairman, US National Intelligence Council
Falls Church, Virginia
January 8, 2019

Preface

The sun was shining on a crisp day in March 2014 as I headed for a meeting at the State Department. After parking my car in a nearby garage and walking just a few blocks, I began having trouble breathing. Because I was a runner, I was perplexed to find myself out of breath. I rested for a few minutes and then proceeded to my meeting. That was Friday. On Monday, I went to see my doctor, who said, "I'm not sure what is wrong, but you need to go to the emergency room." I told her I had some meetings later that day but could work in a visit on Tuesday. My doctor said, "No. I mean now, not tomorrow. We have two world-renowned hospitals within a few miles of my office. Pick one and drive there."

I chose the hospital where my son was born, and it was a good decision. When I arrived at the emergency room later that morning, I waited for less than an hour. A nurse interviewed me, and the doctor decided to give me an EKG to check out my heart. The results came back quickly, and the cardiologist on call said,

"Your heart looks fine. Go home and rest."

"No. I need to know what is wrong," I responded.

The doctor took another look at my files, asked me some more questions, and said, "I really don't see a problem; I am releasing you."

"No," I responded. "I will not leave until you can offer me some alternative hypotheses for what is wrong with me. I also want to discuss what assumptions you are making and whether they are valid."

The cardiologist was not used to patients making such arguments, but realized he was talking to a career CIA analyst who had written books on critical thinking and Structured Analytic Techniques. So, he relented and admitted me for an exploratory procedure the next morning. He said I had "worn him down" to the point he would authorize the procedure despite a mild risk factor. He said he was "90 percent certain" they would find nothing wrong on Tuesday.

My wife came to visit and asked a nurse if she should arrange for my son to drive my car home. She was told by the nurse that the procedure was scheduled for late morning and that I should have no problem driving myself home later that afternoon because I would be awake during the entire procedure and could even watch it on a computer screen.

They did the procedure Tuesday morning, but I did not go home that day. Instead, I was scheduled for major surgery Wednesday morning. Because of that surgery, I am alive today.

Why This Book?

I was a victim of medical misdiagnosis, and I am in good company. According to a report issued in 2015 by the Institute of Medicine, an arm of the National Academy of Sciences, as many as twelve million Americans may be receiving erroneous or late diagnoses every year.[1] This is far more than the estimated hundred thousand deaths per year attributed to errors in hospital treatment. Moreover, the error rate for diagnosing illnesses is likely to worsen as the diagnostic process and health care delivery become more complex.

I began my search for a diagnosis when I started having trouble breathing while running in 2010. It took five years before I finally

1 Erin P. Balogh, Bryan T. Miller, and John R. Ball, eds., *Improving Diagnosis in Health Care* (Washington, DC: National Academies of Sciences, Engineering, and Medicine, 2015).

got a diagnosis following my visit to the emergency room. Over that five-year period, I sought and received treatment from a dozen doctors representing six different specialties—all of whom failed to identify what was causing my problem. I asked many questions during that time and learned a lot about how poorly— and at times, how well—the medical care industry functions in the United States. I condensed these experiences into sixteen actions you can take to improve the quality of your health care:

- Five questions you should always ask your doctor.

- Five obstacles you should expect to encounter.

- Six tips for increasing your chances of getting a solid diagnosis and receiving timely treatment.

I was very lucky. My hope is that people will read this book and live to tell their stories because they applied some of the lessons I learned during my journey.

Design and Content

The book is organized into five chapters with an epilogue and appendices that provide step-by-step instructions for using the techniques:

- The first chapter tells my story, beginning with when I began to detect a serious problem and ending with my emergency hospitalization for major surgery.

- The next three chapters present the key lessons I learned over five years of seeking a diagnosis, learning the value of asking particular questions, anticipating obstacles, and taking advantage of tips.

- The last chapter reveals the correct diagnosis and why I am lucky enough to be here today to write this book.

- The epilogue emphasizes the need to be your own health care advocate.

- The appendices provide step-by-step instructions for how to use six structured techniques that can be applied to most health issues you are likely to confront in daily life.

Interspersed throughout the book are short anecdotes that offer both positive and negative illustrations of each lesson.

Most of the anecdotes were obtained from members of the "5 percent club"—or their close relatives. The 5 percent club is named for those who fall outside two standard deviations of a normal population:

- The lucky members of this club have experienced challenges in getting their conditions correctly diagnosed, took direct responsibility for dealing with their condition, and lived to tell the tale.

- The unlucky members—probably the majority—first tried the standard treatment. When that failed, they tried a second or third treatment. When that failed, they died without ever receiving the correct diagnosis and treatment.

This book contends that people who experience medical problems and recover fall within two standard deviations, or 95 percent, of the area under a standard bell curve (see Figure 1). This is because they self-heal or two or three common treatments cure the problem. However, 5 percent of the population may have more complicated issues, requiring a more thorough diagnosis.

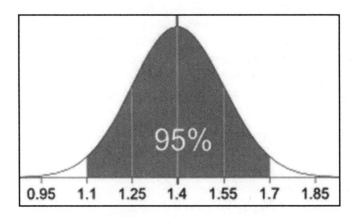

Figure 1. Calculating Two Standard Deviations on a Standard Bell Curve

The thesis of my book is that far more people in this second group would have lived if they had adopted the advice contained in the chapters that follow. I offer this thesis as a hypothesis to be tested and validated or disproved by those much more proficient in medical research.

Disclaimers

My goal in writing this book is to provide a positive—and useful— narrative that will help save people's lives. The intent is to be analytic and not accusatory. I simply want to offer helpful advice. For that reason, I do not refer to any doctors by name, nor do I identify any specific hospitals, medical practices, or facilities.

This is a personal story. Conclusions are presented as testable hypotheses, not proven facts. The author would greatly appreciate any effort by those in academia or the medical profession to document the author's findings and, specifically, to offer additional evidence that would validate—or invalidate—his assumptions regarding patient diagnosis.

The book does not constitute an official release of Central Intelligence Agency (CIA) information. All statements of fact, opinion, or analysis expressed are those of the author and do not reflect the official positions or views of the CIA or any other US government agency. Nothing in the contents should be construed as asserting or implying US government authentication of information or CIA endorsement of the author's views. This material has been reviewed solely for classification.

Acknowledgments

This book has benefited from the contributions of many who have agreed to share their experiences in trying—both successfully and unsuccessfully—to navigate the challenges and peculiarities of the American medical system, including Maryam Allahyar, Kirsti Garlock, Polly Jones, Pamela Noe, Mary O'Sullivan, Kathy Pherson, Kirk Rutherford, Diane Sievers, and Lynda Warren. They would prefer to share their stories anonymously for inclusion in the book, and I have honored that wish, assigning fictitious names to each anecdote. Many also offered valuable advice on how to better focus my story. In addition, I would like to thank Dr. Douglas Boyink, Leanne Cotten, Dr. Mary Edwardson, Cherie Lawson-Shanks, Kristine Leach, Richard Pherson, Danielle Rickard, Dr. Mitchell Ross, and Marie Strassburger for helping me conceptualize the storyline and for providing comments on versions of the manuscript.

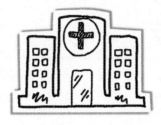

CHAPTER 1

An Undiagnosed Illness

For thirty-five years, I have belonged to a club that runs five miles cross-country over new territory once a week. Thirty to forty of us gather each week without fail. Since joining the club, I have completed over 1,350 five-mile runs. I also ran five Marine Corps Marathons in Washington, DC, recording a best time of three hours and forty-five minutes.

For the first twenty-five years, I had little difficulty keeping up with the pack. Beginning in 2008, however, I started to slow down. I found myself trailing behind. Soon it became obvious that I had become a solid member of an elite group our club calls the "Big behind."

By 2009, I had become frustrated. After running twenty to thirty minutes, I found that my lungs would start to ache. I had to walk to catch my breath before resuming the run. It felt like my lungs could take in only a certain amount of oxygen, and I was forcing them to do more than they could manage. If I pushed too hard, trying to "run through the problem," I would feel a little numbness in my fingers and a slight ache in my upper chest—but nothing serious.

Self-Diagnosis

Could I simply be out of shape? I exercised six days a week. My routine was to run once a week, use an elliptical trainer twice a week (pushing my heart rate to 120-130), and lift weights for forty-five minutes the other three days. I also thought the problem might be that I was overweight. I continued exercising, reduced my food intake, and lost fifteen pounds. Unfortunately, none of these actions made any difference.

I mentioned my frustrations to my family doctor, and we speculated on what could be the problem. Northern Virginia has a high incidence of people with asthma and allergies, so I wondered if that could be the issue. Seasonal allergies were an unlikely cause because my breathing problems were not related to the time of year. I travel frequently and usually enjoy an early morning run in the various cities I visit. In recent years, I had stopped running outside when traveling because running was becoming too strenuous for me.

Is It My Heart?

In 2010, my family doctor and I decided to take more aggressive action. She arranged in February for me to undergo a cardiac treadmill stress test with radioactive fluids to observe the condition of my heart. I underwent testing at a highly credentialed hospital in Northern Virginia with a sterling reputation for dealing with heart disease. A team of three cardiologists reviewed the tests and told me I had scored far above the norm. In March, I did another treadmill test using the Bruce protocol—a maximal exercise test where the patient works to complete exhaustion running on a treadmill as the speed and incline are increased every three minutes. Following the test, the junior doctor on the team thought I could have a problem not getting enough blood to my heart. He suggested I might be a candidate to have a stent inserted into one of my arteries.

The cardiac team decided that I should undergo another test that takes a picture of my beating heart. In December, I had an Echo 20 PW Spectral Doppler heart exam that revealed no significant problems with my heart muscle. The test showed my heart was in good condition—a fact they attributed, in part, to my history as a runner. Once the tests concluded, the senior cardiologist announced that the team reached consensus that my breathing problems were not likely to be caused by my heart. They encouraged me to look for other explanations.

Could It Be My Lungs?

Later in December, my family doctor connected me with a pulmonologist. She tested my lung capacity and found it above average. We discussed the possibility that I might be suffering from exercise-induced asthma or stress-induced asthma. I was doubtful of the first diagnosis because the problem arose only when running and not when doing other exercises. I was concerned that a diagnosis of stress-induced asthma could be correct, as I was feeling some stress managing three companies, traveling extensively, and writing one or two books every year.

My pulmonologist prescribed an inhaler to use just before exercising to see if it made it easier for me to breathe. I started to use it and sensed that it was having only minor impact. My estimate was that it improved my breathing by 10 percent at most. I was prescribed a steroid-based inhaler to deal with my baseline condition as well as a different inhaler to use just before running. Over the course of the next two years, seven different asthma inhalers (first Proventil, then Symbicort and Flovent, followed by Advair, Serevent, Alvesco, and Dulera) were prescribed (see Figure 2).

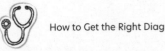

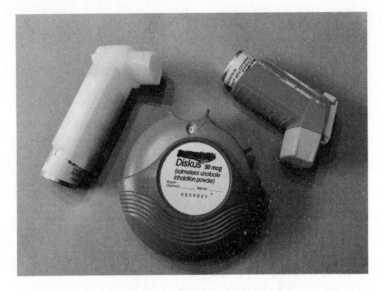

Figure 2. Three of the Many Inhalers Prescribed by Doctors

Symbicort, and possibly Flovent, caused my skin to break out in a "medicinal rash." Little red dots started to appear on my legs and lower trunk. After using the inhalants, the itching was so severe that I could sense it within the soles of my feet and inside the palms of my hands. I went to a dermatologist, who took a biopsy and determined the dots to be a strange form of psoriasis. A patch test established that I had a contact allergy to budesonide, a potent corticosteroid and anti-inflammatory agent found in medicines used to treat asthma, including Symbicort. Other inhalants caused my skin to itch less. I was prescribed a steroid-based anti-itch cream to make the itching more tolerable.

My pulmonologist was puzzled. She did some research to test the hypothesis that I was having an allergic reaction to something in the solvents or suspensions in the inhalers that contained the medication. She failed to identify any such element, however. I continued to use the Alvesco inhaler, which caused the least adverse reaction.

Both my family doctor and my pulmonologist were recreational runners. At one point in my treatment, I suggested that we do a

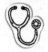

three-mile run together on the weekend, and they could observe how I reacted. Both doctors liked the concept, but, unbeknownst to me, when I proposed some dates, I learned that one of the doctors was a few months pregnant. Although we all agreed the concept had promise, we were not able to make it happen.

Maybe It's Allergies

In January 2011, I went to see our family allergy doctor. My son has a history of allergies. When we took him to the doctor at age four to test him for allergies, he tested positive to 80 percent of the substances. He spent his early life getting allergy shots and continually struggling with asthma, despite being a star forward on a Division One team in the National Capital Soccer League. So, the hypothesis I wanted to test was whether he and I shared some of the same allergies.

My allergy doctor and her senior partner ordered the standard skin prick tests. They came back showing that my only reaction was to some grasses. The fact that I was allergic to some grasses came as no surprise. I had been wearing leggings as a runner for years to guard against that problem as we often ran through high grass. I told the doctors about my experiences with the pulmonologist and the difficulties I had with some of the asthma medications. She prescribed Singulair, an anti-asthma tablet, and continued me on Serevent and Alvesco.

By April, my allergy doctors concluded the medications were not having much effect. They proposed I try a recently developed medication called Xolair. This required a visit to the doctor's office for regular injections. Qualifying for Xolair treatments was a convoluted process. It took over half a year before I could begin my twice-monthly injections.

Moving to the Gold Standard

I told my pulmonologist I seemed to be making little progress. I hoped the Xolair treatments would be the magic solution, but I was skeptical. While we waited for the Xolair treatments to begin, we decided to take the bull by the horns. She arranged for me to see the head of the Asthma and Allergy Center at one of the best nationally acclaimed hospitals in the country.

At our first meeting, the head of the center ordered the standard set of skin prick and blood tests. I told him in advance what the results would be, but he said the center needed to do its own tests. My prediction was mostly correct. I tested positive for the same grasses, recorded a small positive reaction to cockroaches, and negative for everything else. Thankfully, my house and office showed no trace of cockroaches. Allergic reactions to grasses and cockroaches were rejected as contributing to my breathing problems.

The head of the center prescribed Proventil to use when I ran and suggested I conduct a series of self-tests. In phase one of this experiment, he asked me to measure my lung capacity twice a day using a spirometer (a tube you blow into to measure lung capacity) to establish a baseline (*see Figure 3*). I continued to record data for several weeks, entering all the results on an Excel spreadsheet and periodically emailing the results to the doctor.

Pherson Peak Flow Readings, August–September 2011				
Date	Time	First Reading	Second Reading	Comment
25 August	0910	480	500	Walking to work in WDC
26 August	0900	470	480	Walking to work
28 August	1206	320	330	After 1 hour on elliptical
	2130	300	350	After dinner
29 August	0813	370	400	Short trip to Arizona
30 August	0940	530	470	
	2200	440	480	
31 August	0715	400	410	
	2000	540	460	
1 September	0715	450	420	
	2200	500	480	After 1 hour on elliptical
2 September	0645	400	480	Return to WDC
	1045	440	400	
3 September	1100	440	420	Before hiking
	1730	480	460	
4 September	1100	500	480	After exercise
	2300	530	480	
5 September	1000	510	420	Before exercise
	2300	610	530	
Average reading		458	445	

Figure 3. Establishing a Baseline for My Lung Capacity

In phase two, I took the spirometer with me to record my lung capacity every time I ran. My doctor asked me to run until I had to stop and record the time, then record the time when I started to run again, run again until I had to stop and record the time, and repeat this process over the course of the run. At this point in my saga, I could only run at a ten-minute-per-mile pace before I had to stop and catch my breath. Over the course of the following weeks, I conducted the same test but used an inhalant before starting to run.

My guess was that use of the inhaler improved my breathing by 10 to 20 percent. When I checked the data on the Excel spreadsheet, it showed just under a 10 percent improvement on average.

On my second visit to the Asthma and Allergy Center, I suggested that the doctor conduct a "pulmonary stress test" on me. My idea was to strap me up on a treadmill with a few sensors and observe firsthand the difficulty I had running. For some reason, this was never done; one nurse told me that a stress test was often ordered for heart patients, but she was not aware of it being done for those with pulmonary issues. I also asked the doctor if I could be tested for a larger number of allergies, but that was deemed unnecessary. The doctor saw little reason to keep testing, arguing that the treatment would remain the same. I continued to do some self-testing when jogging until our third, and last, session.

At our third meeting, the doctor said that he had concluded that I did not have asthma. He was dismissing me as his patient and recommended that I look somewhere else to find out what was wrong. His specialty was allergies and asthma, and he did not want to comment on issues beyond his specialty. Nor did he want to recommend another doctor for me to see in the hospital. I felt like I had just hit a brick wall at the end of a blind alley.

In January 2012, I began receiving two Xolair injections every two weeks at my pulmonologist's office. I was told it would take at least six months for the treatments to take effect and continued to receive injections until November. My lung capacity was tested on every visit. It always tested well. My self-diagnosis was that the Xolair was causing a 10 percent improvement in my lung capacity at best, but my itchy skin continued to bother me. The good news is that I thought I could run longer (for five minutes) instead of having to stop every two or three minutes.

In October, my pulmonologist arranged for me to have a Helical CT chest scan without IV contrast. In this procedure, an X-ray beam moves in a circle around the body. "Without IV

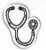

contrast" means that no substance is taken by mouth or injected intravenously (IV) to cause the particular organ or tissue under study to be seen more clearly. The results were negative. The summary report on the scan described it: "No significant axillary, mediastinal, or hilar lymphadenopathy; the heart is not enlarged. There is minimal bilateral lower lobe bronchiectasis; but the lungs are otherwise clear."

My family doctor and I decided in November to drop the Xolair treatments as they were affording little relief. I went back to using the Alvesco inhaler before exercising. Later that month, we decided to submit my case to another asthma and allergy doctor who had served as the personal physician for three presidents and had a superb reputation.

At our first session, the doctor asked if it was okay for two students to observe our consultation and take notes. I thought it was a great idea, thinking they might even contribute some out-of-the-box ideas. The doctor listened to my multi-year saga, and we discussed what alternatives should be considered. He came up with three alternative diagnoses and suggested treatments for each:

1. What if I had asthma in my secondary lung capillaries? He put me on a new medication, Zyflo, to treat this condition, but it did not seem to make a difference.

2. What if the loss of breath was due to sinus drip or acid reflux? He put me on a regimen of Prilosec and Pepcid AC, which ultimately had no perceptible impact.

3. What if I had a vocal cord dysfunction that constricted the amount of oxygen going to my lungs? This would require me visiting an ear, nose, and throat (ENT) doctor for an examination by a different specialist.

I arranged to see an ENT right after the holidays, two weeks before I was scheduled to fly to the Middle East to teach some courses. The doctor ran a laryngoscope down my throat. He saw no thickening and only minor evidence of acid reflux that he assessed as insignificant.

In February 2013, I returned to the allergy doctor who had sent me to the ENT. He recommended that I stop all asthma medications. I did so from February until May. When I stopped the medication, I could run for two or three minutes without stopping, but, by May, I could hardly run at all and usually speed-walked the entire five-mile course—while always looking for short cuts!

In March, my allergy doctor asked me to take a treadmill test to see whether I had restricted breathing problems indoors as well as outdoors (see Figure 4). I did the test on March 10 and encountered the same problems as when running outdoors. I could maintain a fast walk indefinitely but was unable to do a medium jog for more than four minutes. I could not run for more than a minute.

I continued to travel overseas on a regular basis to teach courses on analytic techniques as well as critical thinking and writing skills at various universities, global corporations, and government offices. My travels usually entailed carrying books, instructional manuals, and other course materials in a suitcase that usually weighed over fifty pounds. I recall struggling a little when I had to pull a heavy suitcase up a long hill in Barcelona, Spain, en route to my hotel. That prompted me to start using my Alvesco inhaler again, but it did not make much difference.

In June, while attending a conference in San Diego, I took advantage of the perfect weather to run outside a couple times to see if it was easier in a different climate. I even used the spirometer to monitor my performance, but, despite the change in venue, I experienced no relief.

In mid-August 2013, I stopped using Alvesco or any other long-term inhalant. I tried for two months to run with a spirometer to test whether the breathing problem could be exercise-induced asthma (see Figure 5). I measured my lung capacity about fifty

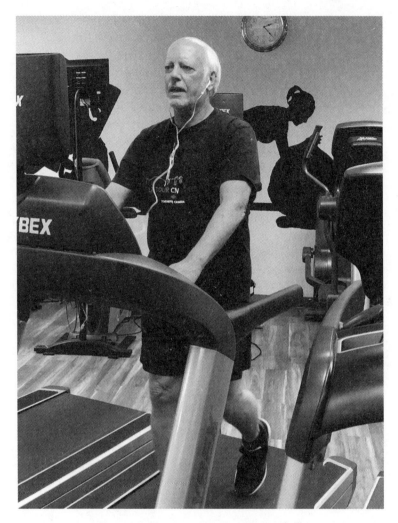

Figure 4. Testing Lung Capacity on a Treadmill

times before, during, and after running, both at home and on business trips to Tucson, Arizona, and El Paso, Texas. I did not record any significant findings, and little changed when I started using the Alvesco inhaler again in late September.

I reviewed my situation with my family doctor. We were running out of specialists to query about my condition. She suggested that I submit my case to the Undiagnosed Diseases Program run by the National Human Genome Institute at the National Institutes of Health and Office of Rare Diseases Research. This would require me to prepare a case history that my family doctor could augment with relevant test results and other paperwork.

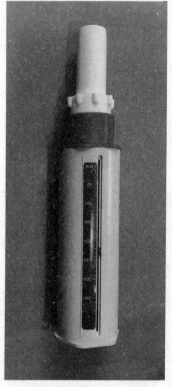

Figure 5. Using a Spirometer to Measure Lung Capacity

If the program agreed to take my case, the process would be to distribute my narrative and test results to a large pool of doctors representing a broad range of specialties who would collaborate in exploring my symptoms and medical test results. My family doctor had used this procedure successfully once before for another patient. It took me a couple weeks to pull all the details into a single narrative (which forms the basis of this chapter). I submitted the application in August 2013. It wasn't until February 6, 2014 that I received confirmation that they had received my letter and would review my application.

In late February 2014, I was back in Barcelona with my wife conducting a Train the Trainers workshop at a local university. After almost a week in the classroom, we spent a day sightseeing. I vividly remember having difficulty climbing a long hill. Halfway up the slope, I turned to my wife and said, "If you did a straight-line projection on my ability to breathe, I think I could be dead in one or two months. Obviously, life does not move in straight lines, so I probably have more time than that, but I really am becoming concerned." To be fair, my condition did not prevent me that day from walking twelve blocks through the Old City while lugging eight bottles of Catalonian wine, which we carried back in our luggage to the United States.

As noted in the Preface, on Friday, March 7, I fell short of breath walking to the meeting at the State Department. I decided that I needed to visit my family doctor as soon as the weekend was over. On Saturday, three other runners in my club and I set out from my home with twenty pounds of flour to mark a five-mile trail that the rest of the runners would follow that afternoon. We were out for over two-and-a-half hours setting the trail. I was able to guide my colleagues on how best to set the course but was having difficulty carrying flour and could only walk, not run. That afternoon, over thirty runners showed up to run the course, socialize afterwards, and celebrate my sixty-fifth birthday.

On Monday, March 10, I went to see my family doctor. She took one look at me, asked a few questions, and told me to drive directly to an emergency room. On the morning of March 12, I underwent major surgery that saved my life.

The next three chapters document the lessons I learned from trying unsuccessfully for five years to get a diagnosis of my condition. My saga involved working with a dozen different doctors representing six different specialties and trying over a dozen different medications. In the process, I learned a lot about the state of medical practice in the United States and what can be done to improve your chances of surviving. If you want to cheat, you can jump to chapter five to learn what transpired at the hospital and afterward.

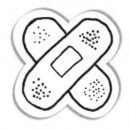

Five Techniques to Spur a Correct Diagnosis

During my five-year odyssey, I noticed a constant tension between the temptation for doctors to start treating the illness versus taking the necessary time to diagnose it. Usually, the default was to treat. In general, this strategy usually turns out to be successful because of the following:

1. In a high percentage of cases, the human body will eventually cure itself. If you visit the doctor, a treatment is usually prescribed, but, at best, it may only be expediting the recovery process.

2. Most illnesses can be treated successfully with just one or two treatments.

But what if the problem is more complicated? Given such strong incentives to treat *and not diagnose*, many of us who have unusual and hard-to-diagnose conditions become frustrated. Our lives become littered with unending visits to doctors' offices, myriads of tests, and a series of unsuccessful treatments. If we die, no one usually will notice that our illnesses were undiagnosed. Our families are grieving; they already knew there was a problem and usually feel impelled to just move on.

What tools or techniques are available to this minority of undiagnosed patients, whom I call the forgotten "5 percent?" How can they get the attention they deserve? This chapter presents six Structured Analytic Techniques (SATs) they can employ to focus more attention on the need for a diagnosis.[2] It describes when the techniques are most useful, what cognitive biases they help to correct, and how they were—or could have been—used in my case. The book also contains examples of how these SATs were used correctly with good results, as well as examples when they were not applied—with serious negative consequences for the patient.

SATs were developed in the late 1990s to provide more rigorous, transparent, and collaborative methods for analyzing a problem, resolving differences, innovating solutions, and anticipating the future. The techniques have proven highly effective in supporting the analytic process in the intelligence community as well as in the corporate world.[3] They are a subset of a variety of practices in the intelligence community that can—and have been—adapted to the medical profession to reduce errors and improve the quality of health care (see Figure 6).

SATs came into prominence following the terrorist attacks on September 11, 2001, and the flawed 2002 National Intelligence Estimate on weapons of mass destruction in Iraq as a way to improve the overall quality of analysis in the US Intelligence Community. Over the years, use of the techniques has spread to other parts of the US government, foreign intelligence services, major corporations, and academia.

The techniques have universal value and utility. Analysis of Competing Hypotheses (ACH), for example, is similar to differential diagnosis in the medical profession.

---

2   A primary source describing SATs as well as when and how to use them is by Randolph H. Pherson and Richards J. Heuer Jr., *Structured Analytic Techniques for Intelligence Analysis*, 3rd ed., (Washington DC, CQ Press/SAGE Publications, 2021)

3   A description of the origins of Structured Analytic Techniques and their role in the analytic process can be found in Randolph H. Pherson and Richards J. Heuer Jr.'s "Structured Analytic Techniques: A New Approach to Analysis" in *Analyzing Intelligence: National Security Practitioners' Perspectives*, 2nd ed., eds. Roger Z. George and James B. Bruce (Washington, DC: Georgetown University Press, 2014).

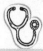

The following key practices or concepts in intelligence analysis have the potential to help medical professionals reduce error rates:

- Recognize how mental mindsets and past experiences can bias a diagnosis (Cognitive Bias and Intuitive Traps).

- Develop more than one explanation for an illness during the initial diagnosis (Multiple Hypothesis Generation).

- Challenge preconceived notions generated by a patient's appearance, age, or race (Key Assumptions Check).

- Focus on disconfirming evidence to quickly eliminate incorrect diagnoses (Analysis of Competing Hypotheses).

- Seek out and value the opinions of others working the case (Coordination and Peer Review).

- Know when to expect deception (Deception Detection).

Figure 6. Intelligence Tradecraft for Medicine

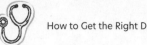

In this chapter, we discuss how you can leverage five SATs to gain more knowledge about your condition while helping your doctor make a correct diagnosis. The six techniques are:

1. Multiple Hypothesis Generation

2. Analysis of Competing Hypotheses

3. Indicators Generation

4. Key Assumptions Check

5. Premortem Analysis

6. Structured Self-Critique

Step-by-step instructions on how to use these techniques can be found in Appendices A-F which contain additional information on when to use them, the value added, their relationship to other techniques, and potential pitfalls to avoid.[4]

Multiple Hypothesis Generation: What Is the Range of Explanations for My Condition?

Instead of telling you X is the problem, let's explore several options.

In his book, *How Doctors Think*, Dr. Jerome Groopman argues that the practice of considering alternative explanations for a medical problem is one of the strongest safeguards against making cognitive errors.[5] He quotes one of his colleagues as saying, "I learned to always hold back [and avoid jumping to a conclusion], to make sure that, even when I think I have the answer, to generate a short list of alternatives."

Multiple Hypothesis Generation is a technique for generating multiple alternatives for explaining a particular issue, activity,

4   See Pherson and Heuer, *Structured Analytic Techniques for Intelligence Analysis*, 3rd ed. for a discussion of Multiple Hypothesis Generation, p. 146-154; Indicators, p. 289-304; Key Assumptions Check, p. 132-137; and Premortem Analysis and Structured Self-Critique, p. 211-220.
5   Jerome Groopman, MD, *How Doctors Think* (Boston: Houghton Mifflin Company, 2007), 66.

or behavior. It is a key technique in the analyst's toolkit and is particularly useful when many factors are involved, a high degree of uncertainty exists regarding the diagnosis, and your doctors and/or nurses hold different views.

The technique helps you, your family, and your doctors avoid—or at least mitigate the power of—several analytic traps, including:

- Coming to premature closure.
- Being overly influenced by first impressions.
- Seizing on the first diagnosis or procedure that looks "good enough."
- Focusing on too narrow a range of alternatives.
- Selecting an explanation that replicates a past success or avoids a previous error.

The value of first considering multiple diagnoses can be demonstrated with the case of dementia. Dementia can be caused by a wide variety of illnesses, injuries, and other factors. Narrowing down the type of dementia is critical to successful treatment. Individuals with Parkinson's disease, for example, may have symptoms similar to other types of dementia, but the treatment could be vastly different. The symptoms of dementia can make it hard to pin down the specific type of the disease a patient has.

Failing to identify the type of dementia can result in poor treatment outcomes due to paradoxical reactions (when a medication causes an unexpectedly opposite reaction to what was intended). For example, individuals with a certain type of dementia called Lewy body typically have a paradoxical reaction to benzodiazepine medications such as Valium. When an agitated patient with Lewy body dementia is prescribed a benzodiazepine medication (which is a typical first-line medication for agitation), instead of calming the patient, the effect is to increase the level of agitation. For these reasons, an attentive doctor should first consider a range of possible forms of dementia and then narrow down the diagnosis to avoid prescribing an incorrect treatment.

In some intelligence services, analysts are not allowed to present their conclusions unless they can demonstrate that they have considered potential alternative explanations for what has occurred or is about to occur. This approach is important during diagnosis of a health issue because the simple process of considering alternative explanations forces you and your doctor to focus on all the available data, not just the information or the tests that are consistent with the lead diagnosis.

A key mistake I made at the start of my journey was not to press my doctors to provide me with a list of possible alternative explanations for my condition. A question I could have asked was: Have you examined anyone else with my symptoms? What did you learn in that case?

Perspective: Persistence in Seeking More Than One Explanation Pays Off!

Nancy's back was killing her, and, after four doctors and multiple tests, she still did not know why.

I developed a nagging ache in my back, toward the center of the upper spine just below the shoulder blades, but a bit lower. If I shifted my position, the pain would go away, but only temporarily.

I made an appointment with my primary care doctor, who initially suggested I take a pain reliever. I said no because I wanted first to know why my back was aching. I was determined to find the root cause of the problem before starting treatment. Blood work revealed no clues, and a review of my activities did not yield useful insights. Lacking a better idea, my doctor suggested the pain could be stomach-related.

I made a second appointment with a gastroenterologist, who grudgingly ordered a CT scan, "Only because your family had a history of pancreatic cancer." But the CT scan provided no clues. The gastroenterologist then suggested that my problem could be orthopedic.

The orthopedic surgeon examined my back and found nothing wrong. I kept insisting on a diagnosis, which prompted him to order an MRI with contrast. The results revealed no back issues but revealed a small cyst on the pancreas.

I went to a second gastroenterologist who is an endoscopy specialist. He scheduled a procedure whereby he inserted a tube with a special camera and retractable needle down my throat into the stomach to photograph the pancreas and take a biopsy. My cyst, thankfully, was small and benign. The doctor told me it could be a cause of the pancreatic discomfort, and he wanted to redo the procedure in two years. When I asked what I should do to get rid of the cyst, the doctor responded, "Nothing."

I went home and did some research on the pancreas. I learned it functions primarily to produce insulin and do some liver bile management. I concluded from my research that I should eliminate as much sugar as possible from my diet. I significantly reduced my sugar consumption, and the ache eventually disappeared.

Two years passed, and I underwent a second endoscopy. The nurse told me, "Whatever you are doing, keep doing it because the cyst is smaller. Come back in two years and we will check it again."

Another two years passed, and I underwent a third endoscopy. The nurse told me, "We recommend discontinuing these tests. The situation is sufficiently stable. Just keep doing what you are doing."

Did I ever get a diagnosis? No, but the ache left along with the sugar.

When I underwent my first test at the hospital's cardiac center, the question they focused on was much more restricted. In essence, they saw their job as determining whether my heart was healthy.

Ideally, the diagnostic process should have started one step before with a brainstorming session involving my family doctor and me. The objective would be to generate a list of all possible explanations for my condition. For example, a good question to explore with your doctor would be "What is the most common cause of what I'm experiencing, and what's the most serious?"[6] In real life this rarely happens because 1) doctors are too pressed for time and 2) the most obvious treatment is usually the right treatment.

A positive example of how this process should play out occurred when I first met with "the president's allergist." At that stage of my journey, I had met with several other allergists and had grown tired of the standard testing procedures. For that reason, I was quick to show the doctor my previous test results and challenge him to come up with some nonstandard alternatives. After some reflection, he generated three ideas, and we implemented a plan for determining if any of them were valid.

One factor may have spurred the doctor to pursue this relatively unorthodox approach. When I first met him in his office, two student interns accompanied him. The doctor asked if I had any objection to them listening to our conversation and taking notes. I liked the concept as four heads are always better than two. Moreover, my visit provided the interns with several important teaching points:

- Listen carefully for information that might suggest a medical history that is not "normal."

- Resist the temptation to come to premature closure.

6   Nudson, Rae. "The Smartest Questions to Ask Your Doctor: What to bring up to be a more informed, proactive patient," *Medium*, March 6, 2019. Accessed March 31, 2019, https://medium.com/s/story/the-smartest-questions-to-ask-your-doctor-b12757820524.

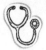

- Make a list of multiple possible explanations at the start of the diagnosis.

Analysis of Competing Hypotheses: Look for Data That Is Inconsistent with the Diagnosis

How would I know which explanation is most likely not true and can be eliminated?

If you ever watched *House* on television, you would have seen many occasions when Dr. House would gather his medical team around a whiteboard, list the potential diagnoses across the top of the board, list the relevant test results and other information down the left side, and then check off which data was consistent—or inconsistent—with each diagnosis. The doctor would then order additional tests to generate additional data. Additional tests would allow the team to dismiss candidate diagnoses until only the correct diagnosis was left standing.

I always wondered to what extent *House* mirrored what actually happens in hospitals. I wished it were an accurate rendition, but knowing the time pressures present in the industry, I have my suspicions.

Dr. House was using a technique similar to a method many intelligence analysts use. Analysis of Competing Hypotheses (ACH) involves generating a complete set of hypotheses (or potential diagnoses), the systematic evaluation of each based on the available evidence (or symptoms and test results), and the selection of the hypothesis that best explains the condition based on evidence that tends to disconfirm rather than confirm each hypothesis (the diagnosis). In essence, the technique focuses attention on which explanations—or diagnoses—can be dismissed because of compelling inconsistent evidence, leaving the "last man standing" as the most likely explanation.

A similar process often used in the medical profession is called differential diagnosis. A differential diagnostic procedure is a systematic process used to narrow down the probabilities of a candidate illness to negligible levels by using evidence such as symptoms, patient history, and medical knowledge. A standard differential diagnosis has four steps.[7]

The physician:

1. Gathers all information about the patient, focusing on the symptoms.

2. Lists all the possible causes for the symptoms.

3. Prioritizes the list by placing the most dangerous possible causes at the top of the list.

4. Rules out or treats possible causes, beginning with the most dangerous condition and then working down the list. The physician removes diagnoses from the list by observing and applying tests that produce different results, depending on which diagnosis is correct.

If no diagnosis remains, then either the physician made an error, possibly by originally failing to list a potential cause, or the condition is undocumented.

The ACH technique—or its twin in medical practice, differential diagnosis—works best when there is a robust flow of data and multiple test results to absorb and evaluate. It helps you and your doctors overcome several mistakes, including:

- Accepting information that confirms one's preconceptions or contradicts prior beliefs.

- Being overly influenced by first impressions based on incomplete data.

- Ignoring or discounting information that does not "fit" the lead diagnosis.

- Failing to generate a full set of explanations at the outset.

---

7   "What Is Differential Diagnosis?" *Sharecare*, accessed March 4, 2019, https://www.sharecare.com/health/diagnostic-procedures/what-is-differential-diagnosis.

- Relying on evidence that tends to confirm one's favored diagnosis but is also consistent with other possibilities and therefore has no diagnostic value.

Simultaneous evaluation of competing diagnoses is challenging. To retain five or seven potential diagnoses in working memory and process how each item of information fits with each diagnosis is extremely difficult. ACH overcomes these obstacles by making it easier to enter, sort, and evaluate the data by working through a matrix one cell at a time *(see Figure 7)*.

Patient	Lead Diagnosis	Alternative Diagnosis 1	Alternative Diagnosis 2	Alternative Diagnosis 3
Inconsistency Score				
Symptom 1				
Symptom 2				
Symptom 3				
Test Result 1				
Test Result 2				
Assumption 1				
Information Gap 1				
Other Information 1				

Legend:
II - Very Inconsistent
I - Inconsistent
N - Neutral
NA - Not Applicable
C - Consistent
CC - Very Consistent

Figure 7. ACH Sample Matrix

Use of an ACH matrix also ensures that all the members of the medical team are working from "the same sheet of music" with shared information, arguments, and assumptions. It helps them gain a better understanding of why there are differences of opinion, and it helps depersonalize an argument when serious differences of opinion are present.

Speaking as a developer, user, and proponent of the ACH method, I am always looking for ways to apply it in my personal life. The concept of trying to disprove a diagnosis is a thread that runs through my entire story. I was able to document on my own that I was not suffering from seasonal allergies, and my trip to San Diego indicated that my problem was not specific to Washington DC's geography. Moreover, with a simple five-minute procedure, the ENT doctor eliminated the possibility that my condition was caused by a thickening of my vocal cords.

On the other hand, my efforts to generate unique data to support a differential diagnosis approach were stymied by the failure to get a doctor to run with me. I also failed to convince several doctors to order a "pulmonary treadmill test" to replicate my experience. One reason could be that such a test does not exist—there may be no billing code for a "pulmonary stress test."

My interaction with the allergist who treated several presidents provides another commendable example of how the technique was applied effectively. The overall experience was flawed, however, because the range of diagnoses considered was not comprehensive. This example illustrates a problem that is hard to overcome; doctors must take care not to offer opinions or diagnoses that deal with issues that fall outside their specialties. Doctors, for example, could unduly alarm a patient by suggesting that one of many potential causes of their discomfort may be some form of cancer. This problem could be mitigated by limiting the number of alternatives to the two, three, or four most viable diagnoses, or by stating that cancer is unlikely but impossible to totally rule out in most cases.

Perspective: Acting on Inconsistent Information

The diagnosis was exercise-induced asthma, but why did it happen when Maria was playing only one sport?

I really enjoyed playing point guard on the basketball team but was starting to have a problem with my breathing, especially when the team was under a lot of pressure. I also was on the swim team, where my friend Sally was having the same problem during workouts. Several other swimmers told us their doctors had given them inhalers to use because they were suffering from exercise-induced asthma.

That made sense to me, so I went to see my pediatrician to get a proper diagnosis. I described my experiences playing basketball. One of the first questions the doctor asked me was whether I played other sports. Did I encounter the same problem with my breathing playing those sports? I told him I was a swimmer but did not remember having problems in the pool. The doctor asked me to run up and down the seven flights of stairs in his building and report if that exercise made it difficult for me to breathe. I did and reported no problems.

The doctor told me that being able to run up and down the stairs with no problem was inconsistent with a diagnosis of exercise-induced asthma. He thought a more likely explanation was that performance stress had constricted my vocal cords, narrowed my throat, and made it hard for me to breathe. He recommended some visualization exercises, like focusing on making my hands warm the next time I sensed a breathing problem coming on. The next time I was on the basketball court, I tried the exercises and was fine. Apparently, I had no need for an inhaler.

The doctor told me he had examined several other swimmers who were complaining of breathing problems and were experiencing the same stress performance syndrome. He treated them the same way successfully without any need for an inhaler. When telling my story to friends, I learned that many other primary care physicians had prescribed inhalers in similar situations when they are not needed.[8]

Indicators Generation: Track the Progress of Your Treatment

How would I know which explanation is most likely true and deserves more attention?

Indicators are observable phenomena that are periodically reviewed to help establish which explanations are most viable. In my case, a set of indicators could have been paired with each potential explanation to track over time which diagnosis was emerging as the most likely explanation for my condition. By establishing a set of objective criteria, doctors and nurses could have tracked whether subsequent developments were reinforcing or undermining the various diagnoses.

Indicators provide an analytic baseline for instilling more rigor into the process and enhancing the credibility of the final diagnosis. They can be used to validate the lead diagnosis, alert one to unexpected developments that may focus attention on a less likely diagnosis, and spot emerging trends or anomalies.

The use of indicators can help the medical team overcome—or at least mitigate—several cognitive biases and intuitive traps, including:

- Continuing to hold to an initial diagnosis when confronted with a mounting list of contradictory evidence.

- Basing a diagnosis on weak evidence or evidence that easily comes to mind.

8　Amanda Loudin, "She Was a Triathlete in Great Shape, So Why Was She Breathless, Lightheaded and in Pain?" *Washington Post*, December 30, 2017, https://www.washingtonpost.com/national/health-science/a-triathlete-found-herself-breathless-dizzy-and-cramping-when-exercising/2017/12/29/202a3b18-cb03-11e7-8321-481fd63f174d_story.html?utm_term=.385ea793e6fa.

- Accepting or rejecting someone else's ideas because the doctor or nurse strongly likes or dislikes that person.

- Claiming the key items of information that turned out to be dispositive in making the diagnosis were easy to identify at the start.

When creating a list of indicators, five rules of thumb apply. Indicators should be:

1. **Observable and collectible**, ensuring that the observations are available to the diagnosing medical team.

2. **Valid,** in that they accurately measure or reflect what is being reported.

3. **Reliable,** in that they will be reported in the same way by different people.

4. **Stable,** in that they can be used over time to allow comparable assessments.

5. **Unique,** in that they point to only one diagnosis. This last condition is often the most difficult to achieve.

Perspective: Let Your Body Tell You if the Diagnosis Is Wrong

Shiloh had a diagnosis, but her body was telling her it was not right. She kept pushing until doctors discovered the real cause of her distress.

As a woman in my early forties, I was enjoying a relatively healthy life until four years ago when I suddenly experienced severe shoulder and neck pain, especially in the morning. Initially, I thought I was sleeping poorly and changed my pillow, thinking this would solve the issue. But it was not your normal "slept the wrong way" pain.

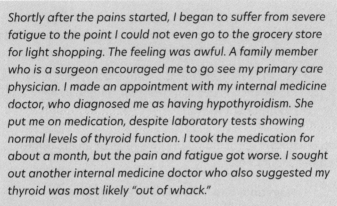

Shortly after the pains started, I began to suffer from severe fatigue to the point I could not even go to the grocery store for light shopping. The feeling was awful. A family member who is a surgeon encouraged me to go see my primary care physician. I made an appointment with my internal medicine doctor, who diagnosed me as having hypothyroidism. She put me on medication, despite laboratory tests showing normal levels of thyroid function. I took the medication for about a month, but the pain and fatigue got worse. I sought out another internal medicine doctor who also suggested my thyroid was most likely "out of whack."

My symptoms were getting worse. I developed excruciating headaches and a feeling of numbness on the left side of my face. I asked myself, "Could it be a brain tumor?" One evening, as I sat on a deck watching deer walk through the backyard with my family member who is a surgeon, he turned to me and asked, "You haven't had a tick bite lately, have you?" I answered, "Yes, about four months ago. It left a tiny dot on my ankle, but I did not get a bull's-eye rash." He put two and two together and said, "Shiloh, I think you have Lyme disease."

I went to an urgent care facility the next day, described my symptoms, and the physician concluded I had Lyme disease. It had to be treated on a long-term basis, and she recommended that I return to my primary care physician for treatment. I did so, but he disagreed with the diagnosis, insisting that my symptoms were consistent with hypothyroidism. Later that week, I was reading a paper when I began to show neurological symptoms—I could not focus or control my eyes. The next morning, I begged my surgeon family member to treat my illness. He treated me for Lyme disease for several months, and now I am disease-free without permanent neurological damage.

In my case, a series of doctors prescribed different asthma medications with the expectation they would address my problem. In total, twelve different medications were prescribed.

The approach was: "Let's see if this one helps. If not, we can try another."

A better strategy, in my view, would be for the doctor to say, "We are giving you an asthma medication. We expect it to have the following effect: it should increase how long you can run without having to stop immediately after you use it by X; it should add a set number of points to the readings you get on your spirometer; and over the next month, it should increase the average amount of time you can run without stopping by Y and over the next three months by Z." The doctor would give me a set of indicators that I could monitor to see if the prescribed medication was doing its job.

Such sets of indicators can be used either to help confirm that a given diagnosis appears to be correct or to signal that the current diagnosis may well be wrong and alternative explanations should be explored. For example, when the lead diagnosis was that I was suffering from exercise-induced asthma, a simple procedure would be to use the spirometer to measure lung capacity before and after I exercised. Similarly, if I wanted to evaluate the viability of a diagnosis of stress-induced asthma, I could have generated a set of indicators that anticipated when I expected to be under stress. As the days progressed, I could then monitor my body to see if these incidents made it harder for me to breathe. If I found no correlation, then the diagnosis was less likely to be correct. In that case, attention should be refocused on finding the real culprit.

Key Assumptions Check: Challenge Your Doctor's Assumptions as Well as Your Own

Could any of the assumptions you are making about my condition and me be incorrect?

Assumptions are something that you accept as true or certain to happen, but without any proof. They are beliefs or ideas that underpin an argument or a diagnosis. Often your doctor will refer to them as "common wisdom." In my company, we often ask students or professionals to list the key assumptions they are making about a situation or event. Invariably, we find that about one out of four assumptions turn out to be incorrect when subjected to critical examination. That is a high error rate, but, in daily life, we often do not notice these errors. We are more likely to focus on the 75 percent of assumptions we make that are correct.

Challenging your assumptions is one of the most important habits you can acquire. If you identify an unsupportable assumption early in the process, you can save substantial time by avoiding going down blind alleys. For this reason, much can be gained by conducting a Key Assumptions Check before you begin to write a paper, pull together a presentation, or try to diagnose what is wrong with you.

An example of an assumption that has been overturned in recent years relates to fatty liver disease. Before 1980, many physicians called it alcoholic fatty liver disease because they assumed consuming too much alcohol caused it. Even if a patient told a doctor he or she did not drink alcohol, the doctor would assume the patient was lying to cover up a bad habit. In 1980, doctors began to recognize the presence of the disease in patients who did not drink. Doctors now differentiate between alcoholic fatty liver disease and nonalcoholic fatty liver disease.

In 2009, the National Institutes of Health (NIH) reported that 20 percent of the US population had one or the other form of fatty liver disease.[9] More recently, the American Liver Foundation estimates that the number of individuals affected by fatty liver disease has increased to 25 percent and it includes many children.[10]

---

9   P. Almeda-Valdes, D. Cuevas-Ramos, and A. Aguilar-Salinas, "Metabolic Syndrome and Nonalcoholic Fatty Liver Disease," Annals of Hepatology 8, no. 1 (2009): S18–24, https://www. academia.edu/20136452/The_metabolic_syndrome_and_nonalcoholic_fatty_liver_disease; and Anna Alisi, Melania Manco, Andria Vania, and Valerio Nobili, "Pediatric Nonalcoholic Fatty Liver Disease in 2009," Journal of Pediatrics 155, no. 4 (October 2009): 469–474, http://www.jpeds. com/article/S0022-3476(09)00568-X/fulltext.

10   "Liver Disease Statistics," American Liver Foundation, October 26, 2017, https://www. liverfoundation.org/liver-disease-statistics/#non-alcoholic-fatty-liver-disease-non-alcoholic-steato-hepatitis.

A Key Assumptions Check is an explicit exercise to list and challenge the key working assumptions that underlie the basic analysis or diagnosis. When the available evidence is incomplete or ambiguous, your interpretation of the symptoms will be influenced by the assumptions you and your doctors make. By critically examining these assumptions and making them explicit at the start, you can:

- Increase your understanding of the basic dynamics at play.
- Uncover hidden relationships as well as links between assumptions.
- Generate new ideas and perspectives.
- Reduce the chances of surprise should new information render old assumptions invalid.

Conducting a Key Assumptions Check can help mitigate against several powerful cognitive biases such as Satisficing and Premature Closure. Satisficing is pursuing the minimum satisfactory outcome for the moment[11] or, more simply put, selecting the first answer that appears "good enough."[12]

Premature Closure is a form of Satisficing, defined as providing a satisfactory answer before sufficient information can be collected and proper analysis performed. Given the time pressure that doctors are under, they must process the available information quickly and render an opinion on the likely cause of your problem or the most appropriate next steps to take, often within a matter of minutes.

The process of challenging your assumptions can also provide an effective check to counter the cognitive bias called Anchoring. Anchoring is defined as accepting a given value of something unknown as a proper starting point for generating an

---

11 "Satisfice," *Merriam-Webster*, accessed March 4, 2019, https://www.merriam-webster.com/dictionary/satisfice.
12 Katherine H. Pherson and Randolph H. Pherson, *Critical Thinking for Strategic Intelligence*, 2nd ed. (Washington, DC: CQ Press/SAGE Publications, 2015), 55.

assessment.[13] In this case, a doctor may have insufficient data to make a solid assessment and compensates by adopting his or her best guess as the likely diagnosis. The doctor then proceeds to make decisions based on that initial, possibly incorrect, diagnosis. The danger of Anchoring is that once people have come to a conclusion, it is exceedingly difficult to convince them they may be wrong.

Perspective: The Need to Think Before You Treat

The doctors only wanted to test and treat Marie, falling victim to several cognitive pitfalls.

Right after the terrorist attack on 9/11, life was stressful enough. But I had no idea how to manage the large, round, silver-dollar-sized bleeding sores that developed on the back of my hands. I put bandages on them—like you put on a child's skinned knee—but at meetings, someone would gasp when they saw blood trickle out from my bandages and drip onto the conference table. The wounds bled unpredictably like "stigmata."

The first doctor thought I may have been infected with anthrax because there was an anthrax scare after 9/11. He ordered tests, but they came back negative. A second doctor thought I had "impetigo," a bacterial infection of the skin. He started me on an intense course of full-spectrum antibiotics, but the "stigmata" was untouched. The third doctor decided I was a "Catholic" psychosomatic whose religious sensibilities were creating the bleeding. He recommended a psychotherapist. A fourth doctor blamed my laundry detergent for giving me "contact dermatitis" but I was already using unscented, non-phosphate laundry soap. Switching to just plain water changed nothing.

I was rapidly losing faith in the medical system; without any kind of rigorous analysis, each of the diagnoses had been presented within minutes of my explaining the problem. For

---

13   Ibid., 55.

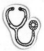

example, why would a "contact" issue involving laundry soap affect only my hands?

The solution presented itself quite by accident. When visiting a goat farm, the proprietor suggested that I read a book on the value of an all-natural diet, more in keeping with what our ancestors ate. One of the book's "takeaways" was to avoid eating processed soy.

This was an epiphany because 9/11 had forced me and many others working in the Washington DC area to forgo sit-down meals because of our jobs. We stocked up, instead, on food bars that contained soy protein. Within a month of eliminating soy-related products, the bandages came off and I could live a normal life again! But whenever I eat a restaurant meal that uses soy, the backs of my hands start to itch or blister the next day.

A Key Assumptions Check can also help you guard against Confirmation Bias. This occurs when additional evidence, information, or test results are seen as confirming the initial conclusion or diagnosis. The problem is that, at the same time, the doctor is less likely to focus on information that is contradictory to the diagnosis, opting instead to ignore or dismiss it.

Taking time to explicitly challenge your key assumptions can help you and your doctors avoid intuitive traps, including the tendency to:

- Project past experiences onto the current case, assuming that the patient is suffering from a condition previously (or recently) treated in other patients.

- Overemphasize small samples by drawing conclusions when insufficient information is available.

- Not take time to consider multiple explanations for the problem.

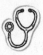

In *How Doctors Think,* Groopman provides a telling example of a doctor who made a bad assumption.[14] The doctor recounts the story of a young man who was brought to an emergency room in the wee hours of the night. He had been found wearing dirty clothes and sleeping on the steps of a museum. He was unshaven and uncooperative when approached by police. The doctor initially assumed he was another homeless hippie who simply needed a good meal and could be sent back out on the street.

After being prodded by an observant nurse, the doctor examined him and discovered he was on the brink of a diabetic coma. The doctor later determined that he was a student who had fallen asleep because he was weak and unable to make it home. His difficulty in responding to the police and the nurses stemmed from the metabolic changes that typified his out-of-control diabetes.

In my case, one of the initial—and incorrect—key assumptions doctors made was that I should be evaluated not as a runner but like any other member of the general population. For example, when I went to the hospital to do my cardiac treadmill test, I noticed that most of the people in the reception room were in much worse physical shape than me. I observed the same dynamic in the reception rooms of the asthma doctors I visited. My test results were evaluated in the context of how I ranked against everyone who had taken the tests. If I had been evaluated, instead, against the population of people who jog or run regularly, I am certain my ranking, when compared to other joggers, would have been much lower than my ranking compared to the general population.

---

14 Jerome Groopman, MD, *How Doctors Think* (Boston: Houghton Mifflin Company, 2007), 55.

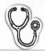

Perspective: Challenging Your Assumptions

Bob had a zest for life until he contracted pneumonia—or was it something more dire?

Bob was known for his dry wit, soft heart, and active lifestyle. At seventy-six, he mowed his own grass, went to Chicago Cubs games, reveled in the athletic successes of his fifteen grandchildren, and drove cross-country to visit friends. Bob had lost his eldest son to cancer and always ended his conversations and emails with "Never Give Up, Charlie," reflecting his strong will and approach to life.

One day, Bob developed a "little" cough that lingered. When he started to lose his breath while taking the garbage out, he went to the doctor, who sent him to the hospital. The doctors in the intensive care unit (ICU) decided he had pneumonia, but no big deal! After a short stay, he was sent home with a portable oxygen tank to ease his breathing. But he failed to improve and had to be readmitted to the ICU.

The doctor's assumption that he had contracted pneumonia was correct, but incomplete. More was going on. Bob was also suffering from a more serious malady: microscopic polyangiitis, which is one of several types of vasculitis, a group of uncommon diseases that result in inflammation of the blood vessels. When the disease affects the lungs and kidneys, treatment must be swift and aggressive. Bob soon needed dialysis, and physicians began to ask if he had an Advance Directive or Do Not Resuscitate (DNR) order. He went into cardiac arrest, and the physicians did resuscitate him. About ninety days after being admitted, Bob died of massive organ failure.

At Bob's funeral, members of his family observed that the medical community had appeared to approach Bob's case assuming he was "a presenting seventy-six-year-old with pneumonia who had lived a good life." A psychiatrist who could read lips came to see Bob shortly before he died. He asked Bob to formulate a sentence with the word "hope." Bob mouthed, "I hope I get better." Sad to say, he did not.

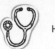

On a positive note, the medical profession is well aware of its susceptibility to cognitive bias and intuitive traps as well as its tendency not to examine basic assumptions. One of the best antidotes is to involve many specialists from diverse backgrounds and areas of expertise in the diagnostic process. This awareness provides one of the intellectual foundations for the establishment of the NIH's Undiagnosed Diseases Program. Some fifty to one hundred patients are invited annually to the NIH Clinical Center in Bethesda, Maryland, to receive a thorough evaluation and engage in consultations as part of the program.[15] These patients are often the lucky members of the "5 percent club."

A key factor in the success of the NIH program is that doctors are encouraged to challenge each other's assumptions in a nonthreatening, collaborative environment. The purpose is not to advance anyone's reputation in the profession, but to come up with a proper diagnosis that had previously escaped discovery and required more imaginative or systematic thinking.

Premortem Analysis: Ask, "What if We Are Spectacularly Wrong?"

If six months from now, you had to explain why I died, what would you say?

Many of us are familiar with the concept of a postmortem. The purpose of a postmortem is to review the historical record and evaluate where and why things went wrong. This usually is a prolonged and painful process that can consume considerable resources. Gary Klein wrote an article in the September 2007 *Harvard Business Review* that poses a brilliant question:

"Why not conduct a premortem type of exercise before we publish our paper or implement our decision to avoid having to initiate a much more embarrassing and labor-intensive process after the fact, should we have turned out to be wrong?"[16]

---

15   For more information on the program, go to https://rarediseases.info.nih.gov/Undiagnosed.
16   Gary Klein, "Performing a Project Premortem," *Harvard Business Review*, September 2007, https://hbr.org/2007/09/performing-a-project-premortem.

Perspective: An Intuitive Premortem Analysis

The doctors wanted to discharge my son Alex from the hospital, but his pediatrician, concerned that their diagnosis could be wrong, vetoed the decision and saved his life.

My son was just recuperating from a bad cold when he and several others were thrown into a heated swimming pool on a cold May evening before the group's confirmation at our church the next day. On Monday after school, he was doing his homework as usual, but suddenly he disappeared. I thought nothing of it, but when I went to get him for soccer practice, he was lying in bed and said he felt "weird," like his "legs were warm on the sides and cold on top." He had a fever, but his hands were icy cold, an odd symptom that had not shown up in my experiential "mother's manual." I figured he was having a relapse and feared a recurrence of the asthma that had resulted from his cold the week before. Opting for caution rather than seeing if he would just "sleep it off," I called the after-hours number for the pediatrician. The on-call nurse practitioner told me that one of the doctors was fortunately still in the office and could see us.

After carefully examining my son for almost an hour and asking if minuscule dots on his chest had "been there before," the doctor arranged for us to be admitted immediately to the hospital emergency room. He was concerned my son had something far worse than the flu. When we arrived at the hospital, they ordered a spinal tap to test for bacterial meningitis, which could be causing the beginning of sepsis and could have been contracted from the warm pool water two days earlier.

My husband picked up our daughter and drove to the hospital. Their entry to the emergency room was blocked by a long ribbon of yellow tape. The security guards told them no one could cross the line because the facility was quarantined. My husband said, "My son is in there," and they

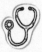

asked my husband for his name. When they heard it, they told him, "You are allowed to proceed."

It felt like an eternity waiting for the results of the spinal tap, but my son's fever had broken, so we were hopeful. At about two in the morning, we received good news: the test was negative! The ER doctor was preparing to release us when we learned that our pediatrician had called in to check on our son's status.

Our doctor's concern was this: What if the diagnosis was wrong? He knew that bacterial cultures from the spinal tap fluid can take two or three days to show positive results and that my son was still at risk. In the worst case, how could he explain why my son died suddenly after medical personnel decided all was well? Our son's pediatrician insisted that the emergency room doctor begin a heavy dose of intravenous antibiotics as if our son had bacterial meningitis or some similar, highly dangerous infection. He also demanded that we be in his office the next day so he could chart out a follow-on course of oral antibiotics.

We never got a definite diagnosis of meningitis, but simply were told that he had contracted some form of virulent virus. My son returned to school after a couple weeks, but it took many months before he could attend a full day of school without naps in the nurse's office. Although the aftereffects of this episode have affected him for many years, our doctor's attentive intervention almost certainly saved our son's life.

In *How Doctors Think*, Groopman describes how one of his colleagues, Dr. Karen Delgado, a specialist in endocrinology and metabolism, has intuitively adopted this approach.[17] She relates that when she was an intern and would admit a patient with what seemed to be a clear and obvious diagnosis, she would ask herself, "What if we are wrong? What else could it be?" Sometimes, she could rearrange the data in her mind to come up

---

with a credible alternative diagnosis that was also consistent with the patient's symptoms. If she could not come up with an alternative diagnosis, she could be more confident the original diagnosis was correct.

A Premortem Analysis is conducted to assess whether a key decision, diagnosis, or action could turn out to be spectacularly wrong.[18]

A Structured Self-Critique is a systematic procedure that an individual or a small group can use to identify similar weaknesses in its own analysis or recommendations. Both should be conducted midway through the diagnostic process, just as the doctor or the medical team is starting to converge on a single, most likely diagnosis. Premortem Analysis involves brainstorming, which is more of a right brain or intuitive process. Structured Self-Critique is a more left-brained, analytic process involving checklists.

The primary purpose of these techniques is to reduce the chance of surprise and the subsequent need for a postmortem should the diagnosis prove wrong. It helps the doctor or medical team identify potential sources of error that may have been overlooked. Two creative processes are involved:

1. **Reframing the issue.** The exercise typically elicits responses that are different from the original ones. Asking questions about the same topic, but from different perspectives, opens new pathways in the brain.

2. **Legitimizing dissent.** Members of a group will often not speak out if they think most of the group would not agree with them. With Premortem Analysis, all the members of the group are asked to come up with a positive contribution to the session by identifying weaknesses in the previous analysis.

---

18 In Structured Analytic Techniques for Intelligence Analysis, Randolph H. Pherson and Richards J. Heuer, Jr. adopted Klein's concept and expanded it into a more robust two-stage process involving right-brained Premortem Analysis and a left-brained Structured Self-Critique.

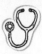

A major benefit of the technique is that it empowers those who have unspoken reservations (for example, a nurse who has just joined the team) to speak out in a context that is consistent with perceived group goals. The approach embraces two different methods to explore all the ways a diagnosis could be incorrect, using a totally unbounded as well as highly structured process.

By legitimizing dissent, the technique offers a strong defense against the perils of Groupthink. Groupthink usually is defined as choosing the option that most members of the group agree with or ignoring conflict within the group due to a desire for consensus. It also protects doctors, the medical team, and their institutions against the Vividness Bias, which involves focusing attention on a single vivid scenario or diagnosis while other possibilities or potential alternative hypotheses are ignored. Vividness Bias can also come into play if the doctor is deluged with promotional materials and media advertisements for medicines that treat a particular ailment. As a result, doctors could become more susceptible to asking if their patients suffer from an ailment that gets a lot of public attention.

An intuitive trap that Premortem Analysis helps correct is Relying on First Impressions (defined as giving too much weight to first impressions or initial data, especially if they attract our attention and seem important at the time).[19] This is a trap that is hard to escape, given the current state of medical care in the United States. Doctors are under extreme pressure from the insurance industry to make decisions as quickly as possible to keep costs (as measured by a doctor's time) to a minimum.

In my case, I believe my primary care doctor intuited the value of a Premortem Analysis and Structured Self-Critique when she recommended that I submit my case to the NIH. The NIH Undiagnosed Diseases Program replicates many aspects of the Premortem Analysis and Structured Self-Critique in spirit, albeit with a different structure.

---

19   Katherine H. Pherson and Randolph H. Pherson, *Critical Thinking for Strategic Intelligence*, 2nd ed. (Washington, DC: CQ Press/SAGE Publications, 2015), 55.

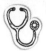

A key challenge to conducting a Structured Self-Critique is making time in a busy doctor's schedule to review an appropriate set of checklists. Even more difficult is finding the time to get a "team" together to conduct a Premortem Analysis brainstorming exercise. At a minimum, a partial solution would be to have doctors take a few minutes at the end of an appointment to ask themselves, "What are the consequences if my diagnosis is wrong, and how could a wrong diagnosis have happened?"

Not only are there logistic hurdles to using these techniques, but doctors are also reluctant (for appropriate legal and other business reasons) to engage in discussions that fall outside the "lanes in the road" of their specialty. They focus on issues that fall within their specialty and are unwilling—for good reason—to speculate about possibilities that could fall outside of their discipline.

I encountered this reluctance several times in the course of my saga. I understood the doctors' logic and the concerns about legal liability but wondered if the system of medical care that many of us now live with in the United States is failing at a fundamental level. If doctors are forced by the system to focus only on what falls within their specialty and avoid the far more fundamental question of what could be wrong with the patient, then we are in serious trouble.

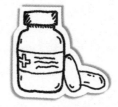

CHAPTER 3

Five Obstacles to Anticipate

One of the most important keys to obtaining a correct diagnosis and effective treatment is to get your doctor intellectually engaged in coming to a better understanding of your condition. In today's world, this has become a major challenge. Doctors—as well as everyone else on the doctor's staff—are under severe time pressure to move patients through the office as quickly as possible.

A typical—and efficient—office has several rooms in which to park patients as information is gathered. Often you will see flags or other colored cards outside the door to signal how far along the patient is in the interview process, with the last color signaling to the doctor that all preparatory tasks have been performed and the patient is ready to see him or her. In the United States, usually no more than fifteen minutes is allocated for this doctor-patient exchange.

This assembly-line production process places a premium on minimizing the time a doctor spends on diagnosing the problem. Such time pressures can also discourage the practice of seeking the views of other doctors and nurses or to brainstorm potential strategies with them in a group setting. The imperative instead is to come to closure quickly on required testing and implement a treatment regimen. In Chapter 3, we present five manifestations of this phenomenon and discuss the best ways you as a patient can overcome them. The five obstacles are:

1. A short time window to see the doctor.

2. The tendency to treat conditions in a serial fashion.

3. The tyranny of specialization.

4. The failure to diagnose.

5. The reluctance to engage and discuss your condition with other doctors.

Short Appointment Time Windows

I have only fifteen minutes to see you.

As noted above, to maintain a profitable practice, doctors normally plan to spend no more than an average of fifteen minutes with each patient. In order to meet this target, doctor's offices have adopted a set of standard practices to make the processing of patients as efficient as possible. These practices include having patients fill out forms before coming to the office; sending text or phone messages to confirm appointments and ensure patients arrive on time; processing payment before the session; and having a nurse practitioner or another member of the doctor's team conduct an initial screening that may involve taking your temperature, checking your blood pressure, updating your list of medications, and asking about allergies. All the information collected from the patient is then gathered in a folder for the doctor to peruse before he or she walks into the room to see you. These practices make a lot of sense and can substantially reduce how much time a doctor needs to spend with you.

I vividly recall waiting for three months before I could see the ENT doctor to learn if an abnormal thickening of my vocal cords caused my breathing problems. I had already visited almost a dozen doctors seeking a diagnosis and was hoping this visit could be the silver bullet, out-of-the-box solution to my problem. Several weeks before the much-awaited appointment, I contracted an ear infection that was proving resistant to the normal treatment of antibiotics my family doctor prescribed. This prompted us to consider whether I should have a tube inserted into the eardrum to ensure proper drainage.

From my perspective, the long-awaited visit to the ENT provided the opportunity to "kill two birds with one stone." I might discover a reason for my shortness of breath and decide on the proper treatment for my ear infection in one appointment! Unfortunately, I was mistaken.

As it turned out, the doctor was running late. When he came to my room, I raised both issues with him. He decided to look at my ear first. We reviewed the record of already going through two treatments of antibiotics, and he recommended trying an even stronger dose before installing a tube. I agreed and then asked him about my throat. He responded, "My last appointment took more time than was scheduled, and I have already used up the ten minutes I can spend with you. Take the medicine and come back in two weeks. When you come back, I will then look at your throat. I don't have the extra five or ten minutes to spare to do that now."

Needless to say, I left the office extremely frustrated. Over a ten-minute period, we had managed to come up with a good strategy for dealing with my ear, but I had completely failed to learn anything about the thing I really cared about—which was my breathing problem. At first, I was exasperated. But later that week, I realized the doctor's response made sense. I would have to come back in two weeks, regardless, to have my ear checked out, and waiting two more weeks to learn if my throat was the source of my condition was not unreasonable. I had been chasing after this problem for three years, so what was the relative cost of waiting another two weeks? Moreover, my doctor could have been just as frustrated as I was that the system did not allow him to take more time with me in the office (I later learned that this was the case).

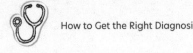

Two years after my major surgery, I had a different experience. I was visiting a doctor for the first time since the surgery. We were wrapping up my fifteen-minute appointment, and I mentioned that I planned to write this book. He liked my approach to the book and sat down to discuss some key themes. I told him I was surprised he could take an extra fifteen minutes just to talk to me. He said he recognized the need to spend quality time with patients and tried to plan for this accordingly. We had a great conversation.

As I departed, I observed that, in addition to the desk where I had signed in, there was another reception desk across the hall that I had not noticed when entering the office. That reception desk was dedicated to those who had come to the doctor's office for cosmetic surgery. Cosmetic surgery is much more lucrative than traditional medical practice because patients usually pay in cash, and the doctor can avoid the bureaucratic costs of processing insurance claims.

My hypothesis, which I never validated, was that the doctor (to his credit) had established the cosmetic surgery practice in part to relieve some of the monetary pressures—and time constraints—he faced with his more traditional medical practice.

My advice for dealing with the fifteen-minute window is not to complain about the short amount of time a doctor can spend with you, but to be prepared to take maximum advantage of the session. In addition to the tips listed in the next chapter, decide how you want to organize the time you will spend with your doctor. For example, one technique is to write down a list of questions you want to ask and give your doctor a copy to help structure the discussion *(see Figure 8)*.[20]

---

20   See Groopman, *How Doctors Think*, 260–264, for an illuminating discussion of the importance of asking your doctor questions.

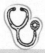

Questions you might want to ask your doctor:

1. Have you had a good day so far?

2. Did you get my list of medicines and questions I want us to address today?

3. Could the change I just mentioned in my activities, behavior, or diet have caused the problem?

4. If your lead diagnosis is correct, what should I expect to experience in the coming days (confirming the diagnosis)?

5. What might I experience in the coming days that would be inconsistent with your diagnosis (suggesting a new diagnosis may be needed)?

6. What are some of the alternative diagnoses you are considering? What else could it be?

7. Could I have more than one problem?

8. Can I keep some records or generate some new data that would help you track my progress? Would it help if I documented my response to the proposed treatment?

9. The negative test results just don't make sense. Should we consider retesting?

10. Is there anything else you recommend that I do?

11. How long would it take before we should consider a different treatment or diagnosis?

12. Would there be value in seeing a doctor in another specialty?

Figure 8. A Dozen Questions to Ask Your Doctor

An even better strategy is to give the list to the nurse before you see the doctor. The list might spur the nurse to ask more probing questions and include additional useful information in the folder he or she will give the doctor. If there are routine lab tests that you know will be needed, call the nurse and arrange to take the tests in advance so the results will be available when you meet with the doctor.

When meeting with your doctor, be alert to whether the doctor is asking open-ended questions that give you space to explain all the aspects of your condition. Is the doctor really listening, or is he or she only focused on what would be the most likely diagnosis or best treatment to suggest? Does your doctor want to know what really bothers you the most? How would your doctor react if you asked, "Do you have time for me to tell you my story?"

Perspective: Beware of Too Much Treatment

Helen's quality of life was crashing; what could turn this around?

My mother Helen, at age eighty-eight, suffered from poor quality of life, dealing with chronic arthritis and other debilitating conditions. After one Thanksgiving dinner, I contacted my brother, who was out of town, suggesting he visit her in the next few days because I did not think she would last much longer. She continued to hang in there, but such episodes occurred several times for the next two years. The deterioration seemed to coincide with the decision to increase her medications.

My mother had a DNR order in place, and I had power of attorney for her health care. As her quality of life was failing quickly, my brother and I decided to take her off all medications except for three the doctor considered essential: her blood pressure pill, a small dose of a thyroid medication, and an anti-depressant that she had been taking for years.

Within three months, my mother was nearly a new person. We could not fix her arthritis, but her mind was back, she looked better, and she had a much-improved appetite. We were thrilled! She lived another five years in relatively good health and good mind for someone who passed away at ninety-three.

A key consideration is how a doctor tries to relate to you. Does the doctor come across as the font of all knowledge who spends most of his or her time talking, with you playing the role of the supplicant? Alternatively—and preferably—is the doctor working with you to discover what is causing the problem and spending most of his or her time listening? As Dr. Atul Gawande, a Boston surgeon and author of *Being Mortal* argues, "Doctors, clinicians, and their patients should sit together, not across from each other."[21]

Serial Treatment

Let's try treatment A; if that does not work, we will try treatment B; if that does not work, I am sure treatment C will do the trick!

In most cases, after a doctor has been presented with a detailed set of symptoms, the most obvious and best course of treatment is clear. The doctor probably has seen many similar cases in the past, and invariably the treatment prescribed is effective. This strategy—to prescribe a treatment that best matches the problem and wait and see if it works—also saves the doctor time. He or she does not need to devote time to considering alternative diagnoses, and the chances are good the treatment will work. If the first treatment fails, then the chances are even better that a second treatment will work. The dilemma for a time-pressed doctor then becomes: at what point do I stop proposing treatments and spend time (usually unbillable) trying to diagnose the problem?

21   Atul Gawande, "Being Mortal's Villages: The Value of Community and Choice as We Grow Older," live-streamed conversation, Beacon Hill Villages Event, Temple Rodef Shalom, McLean, VA, September 25, 2017.

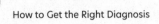

In my case, cardiologists had ruled out a heart problem, and my next set of doctors specializing in pulmonology, asthma, and allergies marched me through a set of inhalers, one at a time, hoping that the next one I tried would work. Some of the inhalers caused side problems such as skin rashes that further complicated the process. Instead of focusing only on what was helping me breathe better, the ancillary problem became the primary concern: which inhaler had the fewest side effects. Unfortunately for me, this process of focusing on the symptoms and not the cause also consumed a lot of my time, extending the time it took to come up with a correct diagnosis. Each time I was prescribed a new inhaler, I would have to "try it out for a month or two" to see if it had a positive impact.

The best defense against the "serial treatment syndrome" is to press your doctor to stop proposing treatments or prescribing medicines and focus more energy on diagnosing the problem. Ideally, attention should focus from the start on getting a proper diagnosis, but this usually is not the case. If the first treatment proves ineffective, most doctors will be sensitive to patient complaints that a process of serial treatments could be wasting a lot of the patient's time.

Tests that generate false negative results pose a real challenge for the medical profession. An ER doctor told me that as many as one in five tests he sees for cardiac and knee problems turns out to be a false negative. Rarely does a doctor tell a patient, "Your test result was negative, but the chances are one in five that there really is a problem." If a patient gets a test that says there is no problem, most patients will find it even harder to say to their doctor, "I know the test results are negative, but something still is wrong." As one doctor said, patients should have enough courage to tell their doctor they have not done enough to solve their problem. And doctors should listen.

Perspective: Engaging Your Doctor as Coach

When they told Julia she was about to die, her doctor helped coach her to a winning solution.

In 1993, I had a mole removed that was an aggressive type of malignant melanoma. My doctor told me there was no chemotherapy or radiation that would touch this, and that I was going to die! My response could best be described as mental paralysis. My doctor proposed to remove a large section of tissue, muscle, and nerve surrounding the mole and lymphatic sections to determine how much the dreaded disease might have spread.

At the time, I was training to climb in the Himalayas. It was the trip of a lifetime, and it could be the last trip of my life. I was not about to miss it. I was in great physical shape, had a daughter who was planning a wedding, and wanted to experience the joy of grandchildren before I died. I told the physician I would not agree to the removal of the lymph node sections. He countered that this was standard protocol. My trip was scheduled for seven weeks after the surgery, and major surgery involving the lymph nodes would prevent me from going. If I was dying, I wanted the lesser surgery, more quality of life, and the trip to Nepal as planned.

My doctor agreed to the lesser surgery. Immediately following the surgery, I began researching everything I could find on natural approaches to curing and preventing cancer. I told my doctor I planned to take high doses of shark cartilage. He immediately recoiled, saying, "I can't prescribe that." I anticipated his response, as it was not an accepted approach in "Western medicine." I then rephrased my statement, saying, "I intend to take high doses of shark cartilage. Do you think it will harm me?" He quickly smiled and said, "No, I don't think it will."

I started taking the shark cartilage and began meditating for a half hour each day (mentally focusing on the classic Pac Man game, where my good cells were eating my bad).

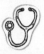

I rollerbladed twelve miles a day and worked out with a Pilates trainer.

I made the trip! The doctor sent my files to a colleague with whom he had trained at Oxford University in the UK. His colleague was in China at the time and would be only an hour away by plane should I get into trouble in Nepal.

I still do all these activities, except for the meditation—and the shark cartilage dose is much smaller. That was twenty-four years ago. If I had gone home after first hearing my diagnosis, laid down on the couch, and believed that I was going to die, I feel I probably would have. Life is too precious! We all know our own wills and our bodies. One must be proactive to enhance the possibilities of good medical outcomes.

The medical profession, however, has one major advantage on its side. Several doctors who have treated me have said that as much as 80 percent of the problems they encounter are likely to go away on their own over the course of time. Treatments may accelerate the healing process or make the patient feel more comfortable, but they may not be necessary. If the patient recovers, it may never be known if the treatment prescribed was the correct one or not.

The Tyranny of Specialization

I can only speak to my area of expertise; it would be inappropriate for me to speculate on matters that lie outside my specialty and could be causing the problem.

American medicine is highly specialized. As my family physician put it, her job is to monitor my health and connect me with the appropriate specialist to deal with problems as they arise. To assume that primary care doctors should be all-knowing is unfair; they are generalists. Their function is to keep you healthy, treat

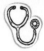

the simpler problems, and look for indicators that something more dire may be afoot.

Doctors also face potential serious legal problems should they offer incorrect medical advice, particularly outside their specialty. Medical malpractice insurance is already astoundingly expensive, and it is a major factor driving up the cost of medical services.

In the United States (and across much of the world), we have constructed a medical profession composed of specialty stovepipes. Each specialty operates within its own walls. Minimal collaboration takes place across those boundaries.

Over the course of my five-year journey, I specifically recall talking to doctors working in three different specialties who told me that they were confident my problem was not relevant to their specialty. They said their conclusion was based on their personal observations, their analysis of my symptoms, test results, and my failure to respond positively to prescribed medications. When I then asked what I should do next, I was frustrated by all three answers I received.

1. The first doctor suggested I set up an appointment with my family doctor to explore other options. That made sense to me, but I was frustrated he did not suggest any paths to pursue.

2. The second doctor helped me test and eliminate four different potential diagnoses that fell within his sphere of his expertise but was reluctant to speculate on what other doctors might find.

3. The third doctor, who worked at a medical institution with an international reputation for treating individuals with difficult cases, told me categorically that my problem was not related to his specialty and released me as a patient. I asked whom he thought I should talk to next in the institution to find out what was wrong with me. He said simply that he could not recommend any doctors outside his specialty. When pressed, he said

I might seek out a doctor in a specialty I had yet to try, but would not make a specific referral. The doctor who referred me to this institution was as shocked as I was by the response and the reluctance of the institution—as well as its doctors—to take some responsibility for treating me as a whole person.

Unfortunately, this obstacle is not easy to overcome. Perhaps the best strategy is to have a family doctor who is adept at helping you traverse the various specialties as you embark on your quest for correcting your condition. Some doctors may prove more willing to offer advice on new paths to explore than others. And in some practices and institutions, you may discover that this does not prove to be a problem at all.

Perspective: Bouncing from Specialist to Specialist

Ron's fingers were swollen and really hurt, but five doctors could not come up with a correct diagnosis and treatment.

One day, I noticed swelling and pain in two fingers—one on each hand. When it became noticeable to others and was affecting my sleep, I went to see an orthopedic physician's assistant (PA) who had resolved a previous hip problem. The PA was shocked by the swelling. He gave me a steroid shot and prescribed indomethacin. It had knocked out a previous case of gout, so I left feeling confident. When I did not get better, the PA then prescribed prednisone, did a thorough arthritis panel blood test, and took X-rays.

Soon more fingers started to swell, and the pain level increased. I was prescribed another pain medication and referred to a rheumatologist. She reviewed my blood test, prescribed Methotrexate, and increased the dose from two to eight pills a week. She prescribed different medicines and injected a steroid into the affected fingers, but the relief quickly wore off. Having had little success, she directed me toward "the best hand guy in town."

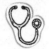

This orthopedic hand specialist took X-rays and offered me three choices: joint replacement, which he did not recommend because of the number of joints; cutting the nerves in all five fingers, which would relieve the pain but also render them useless; and taking two doses of Aleve twice a day forever. After rejecting the choices, I visited my rheumatologist, who prescribed Humira—a highly effective injectable I could self-administer. She also prescribed pain relief, but I had her reduce the dosage to avoid the risk of addiction. The Humira did not work, so she ordered an MRI. I learned that Humira is for rheumatoid arthritis and psoriatic arthritis, both of which I did not have. I asked if I had osteoarthritis. She did not know but told me to stop taking Humira.

I checked back with my first doctor, who referred me to a neurologist who tested me for carpal tunnel syndrome. My test results were the worst he had seen in thirty years, and he recommended surgery on my right hand only, to keep one hand semi-usable. After the surgery, some of the numbness went away, but the pain and swelling remained. The surgeon said, I was "more than welcome to have someone else quarterback" my treatment.

My hands continued to worsen. When my family moved to a new city, I picked a highly respected rheumatologist to seek a diagnosis and treatment. On seeing my hands, she exclaimed, "Oh my God!" She used a Doppler device to look for inflammation, and the results looked like a Category 5 hurricane. She repeated the X-rays, MRIs, and blood test, but came up with no new diagnosis.

Over the course of my medical journey, I had documented all my treatments. I gave my notes to the rheumatologist, who did a thorough eight-page write-up on my case and, at my urging, consulted with her peers—but it was to no avail. Now, after more than twenty-five appointments with five different doctors in various specialties, MRIs and X-rays, the ingestion of dozens of medicines, and surgery, I still have no relief. I thought medical treatment should begin with a

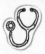
diagnosis, which may require some testing, before leading to a treatment plan. I received some tests, and a lot of treatments, but I was amazed at the relatively small amount of time devoted to coming up with the correct diagnosis.

Brian suffered from a similar condition but solved it on his own.

For several years, I went to many doctors to complain about big, swollen "knots" on my finger joints. The doctors gave me a long list of medicines to take, none of which helped. They just skipped the diagnosis stage, moving right to treatment. The pain got so bad that I gave up playing string instruments, which made me was incredibly sad. When I fell seriously ill after a meal at a Thai restaurant and later, after snacking on a large bag of peanuts on a boat, I realized I was severely allergic to peanut products. I was sixty years old, had never been diagnosed with an allergy, and had been eating peanuts all my life. I gave up peanuts and now I am happily playing all the string instruments that brought me so much joy. I know now when I have been exposed to peanuts or peanut oil because my fingers hurt the next day.

The Failure to Diagnose

Let's run some tests and treat you for what most likely caused the problem. If you get better, it really does not matter what caused it.

Most doctors in the American medical system are paid little to nothing to diagnose your condition. The primary revenue generators in the system are more tangible activities such as office visits, tests, prescriptions, and hospitalizations. A billing code could be set up for diagnosis, but how would an insurance company know if the time billed *thinking* about your case was being spent wisely? Should doctors be required to log their time spent researching articles and books, or placing phone calls to colleagues seeking consult, or time spent on their own deliberating your ailment? What if the doctor merely sat down and thought long and hard about your problem?

Perspective: What if the Obvious Diagnosis Is Wrong?

The pediatric nurse said, "It's only a virus, get over it." But George almost died.

I flew to Washington, DC, for two weeks with my nine-month-old baby to help take care of my mother who was recovering from surgery. I had a happy, energetic baby, but he was becoming more irritable. After a couple days, I noticed he was more lethargic and cried more than usual. He seemed to be peeing more as well and would reach out immediately to grab his bottle when it was feeding time. I started giving him more formula and some apple juice to drink, but he seemed to want more and more.

We were lucky that a pediatrician lived just down the street. She agreed to stop by the house to look at him. After a short visit, she suggested I bring him in for an examination the next morning. I did, and the doctor said it was probably a flu virus. She told me to take him home and let him work his way through it.

Later that day, my baby became even more irritable; he was crying constantly and could not be soothed. I gave him many bottles, and his diapers were totally soaked through when I changed them. When I called the doctor around four in the afternoon, she continued to think flu was the likely cause. I was urged just to wait it out. By midnight, I was starting to become seriously concerned. My baby's condition kept getting worse, not better. At two in the morning, I called the doctor again. The impatient response was, "Bring him in for another examination in the morning." I got almost no sleep that night.

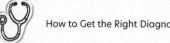

After meeting with the doctor for the second time, my instructions were to "let the virus run its course." By the afternoon, I was totally exhausted. My mother told me to take a walk in the park while she looked after the baby. As I was on my walk, I got a text saying, "Come home now." My baby was limp and had lost all his color. We decided at once to take him to the emergency room.

When we arrived at the hospital, the emergency room doctors saw him immediately. They tested his blood sugar levels, which were well above nine hundred. The team diagnosed his problem as diabetic ketoacidosis (DKA). He was transferred by ambulance to another nearby hospital with better pediatric care and admitted to the ICU.

While they were treating my baby, I will never forget a resident who walked out to tell me, "Your baby is not out of the woods yet. There could be cerebral edema or swelling of the brain, which could be fatal. I need to go back now." A shiver went down my spine; I stood there paralyzed with fear. Subsequently, a nurse came out to deliver a more comforting message: "Good news: he is starting to pink up." Most of the next week was spent at the hospital, learning how to treat a baby with diabetes. My baby recovered with no complications, but it was a close call.

As a result, the process of diagnosing a problem is often seen as ancillary, while other billable activities are deemed to be a higher priority. Most doctors feel obliged to render at least an initial diagnosis, but usually lack the incentives to generate a more thorough diagnosis, much less one that would explore in any depth potential alternative explanations for the condition. Many doctors are also reluctant to reexamine the validity of their original diagnosis because it may require repeating negative tests, adding referrals, or suggesting more invasive tests or procedures.

In a 2015 study by the Institute of Medicine, which estimated that as many as fifteen million American adults are misdiagnosed each year, diagnostic errors are said to occur for a multitude of reasons, making it hard to detect and track them. Some key reasons are the lack of collaboration among clinicians, patients, and their families; the lack of feedback about incorrect diagnoses; and the tendency of the health care industry to discourage transparency and disclosure of errors.[22]

Across much of the medical profession, a default strategy has evolved to minimize time spent on diagnosis and focus instead on prescribing the treatment most likely to be effective. If that fails, proceed with the second-most effective treatment. My suspicion—which I present as a testable hypothesis for medical researchers—is that 95 percent of most medical conditions are cured, successfully addressed, or cure themselves after a patient has gone through two treatment regimens. The remaining 5 percent are the wicked problems or outliers that in statistical terminology fall outside two standard deviations of the norm. It is the members of the "5 percent club" who are at greatest risk of receiving inadequate attention and dying without ever being properly diagnosed.

If this hypothesis is correct, then a case can be made that doctors can expect that 95 percent of their cases are likely to be cured or appropriately addressed without ever being fully diagnosed. Most professionals would be ecstatic if the error rate in their profession was only 5 percent. The problem, however, lies with those of us who fall outside two standard deviations and are members of the "5 percent club." The incentives for grappling with our problems are severely diminished.

A good example of how this process can play out is provided by most of the allergy doctors my family and I have encountered. Usually, the first step is to subject you to a set of six skin prick tests. In my case, I know that I will test positive for several grasses but nothing else. When I tell a new allergy doctor that will be the result, the answer is always that their procedures require that

---

22   Lena H. Sun, "Most Americans Will Get A Wrong or Late Diagnosis At Least Once in Their Lives," *Washington Post*, September 22, 2015, https://www.washingtonpost.com/news/ to-your-health/wp/2015/09/22/most-americans-who-go-to-the-doctor-will-get-a-wrong-or- late-diagnosis-at-least-once-in-their-lives-study-says/?utm_term=.c53bda02450a.

they order a new test. They say they want a lab they trust to run the test and, besides, it is covered by insurance. The results are always exactly what I have predicted. That has led me to wonder if the actual reason for the testing was to help compensate the doctors for time spent thinking about my case and trying to come up with a diagnosis.

Doctors are ruled largely by what the insurance industry allows them to bill. In my search for a diagnosis, I asked several doctors if they could run a "pulmonology treadmill test" to observe firsthand how my lungs were performing as I ran out of breath running on the treadmill. Neither the pulmonologist nor the asthma doctor warmed to the idea. In subsequent years, when I mention this to other doctors and some in the medical industry, they have speculated that the reason could be that there is no code to allow charging for a pulmonary treadmill test.

Reluctance to Team with Other Doctors

I really cannot spare the time to seek out other doctors to compare notes about your condition. Nor am I sure I need them to help me with your case.

Most of the doctors I have encountered are knowledgeable, intelligent, and care about my condition. They have developed substantial expertise after years of academic and residential training and medical practice. Some of the best are highly focused on their particular specialty and widely viewed as standouts in their field. All of these attributes can work to the disadvantage of the patient if they lead the doctor to conclude that he or she does not need anyone else's help to deal with your condition. In fact, a specialist confronts several disincentives for reaching out to other doctors for advice:

- It takes time to arrange a meeting or schedule a phone call to discuss the case.
- If looking for a perspective from someone outside their specialty, they may not know who is best to call.

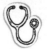

- If they engage someone outside their specialty, they may not be "talking the same language" or making the same assumptions.
- They do not like having to deal with other doctors.
- They believe they are fully capable of dealing with the situation on their own.

As a result, it was unusual for my doctors to converse or compare notes with each other except in one instance. I was lucky enough to have one of my doctors recommend me to another doctor who was a friend of hers. The doctors had a strong social bond and a trusting professional relationship. This made it easier for them to find the time to discuss the progress of my case.

The usual practice was to have my family doctor send appropriate documents to a specialist she had recommended. The specialists, in turn, would send her copies of what they found. This process allowed my family doctor to track my case. In hindsight, I would have benefited greatly if the various doctors engaged in a conference call to brainstorm the peculiarities of my case, particularly when a treatment did not seem to be working. I recognize that such a practice may be difficult to achieve given the time pressures of the profession, but it could end up saving time in the long run if a diagnostic breakthrough is achieved.

The difficulty of getting doctors to collaborate came up several times when I was hospitalized. Nurses who attended me told me they were continually frustrated by how difficult it was to get doctors to talk to each other. In some cases, they had to actively collude among themselves to get doctors working the same case to visit the patient at about the same time. When the doctors arrived, the nurses would block the door or encircle them in the hallway to ensure that they stopped to talk to each other. Another strategy is to get the nurses working your case to exchange information and compare insights on how to best deal with your condition.

Perspective: Failures to Communicate

Miscommunications left Howard abandoned in a deserted wing of a major Manhattan hospital, where he almost bled out.

I had just arrived in New York to teach a course to a well-known consulting firm. As my taxi arrived at my hotel in Manhattan around six that evening, I felt pressure emanating from the lower-right side of my back. The sensation was unmistakable: I knew I was having another kidney stone attack. I asked the front desk to direct me to the nearest hospital. I took a taxi to the hospital and took a seat in the waiting room. I was not admitted to the emergency room until eight, by which time the pain had become excruciating. I was happy the doctor gave me some powerful pain relievers before I was wheeled up to the eighth floor to get an MRI scan to locate the stones.

I had been drinking a lot of water, and, after the MRI scan, I felt a pressing need for relief. The orderly gave me a large plastic jar and wheeled me into a private room that was on the way back to the ER. I relieved myself and waited for someone to come back for me. I always bring a newspaper to the hospital, so I spent the next forty-five minutes contentedly reading the New York Times. I later learned that, about this time, my wife had called the hospital, and the receptionist could tell her little about my status.

After almost an hour-long wait, the newspaper brushed my left arm, and the IV tube came out. My arm started spurting blood. I walked into the hall only to find I was in an almost-deserted wing of the hospital. I could not stop the bleeding and started to panic until I saw someone in scrubs a dozen rooms away. He ran up to help me, stopped the bleeding, and paged an orderly to take me to the ER.

This time, the orderly showed up in less than a minute. As he started to wheel me down the hall, he asked me: 1) Did you come from the north or the south wing of the ER? and 2) What is your room number? I could not answer either

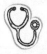

question because, at the time, the pain had totally occupied my attention. When we arrived at the ER, I recognized someone who had been sharing an alcove with me, and I pointed the area out to the orderly. He then informed me that it was my responsibility to remember my room number. I asked him what the room number was. He took a couple steps, pulled back a curtain, and revealed the number seventeen stenciled on the wall. I asked myself, "How could they ever have expected me to know that? I can't see through curtains!"

In hindsight, the ER staff and the MRI staff were obviously not communicating. For almost an hour, a major Manhattan hospital had lost a patient who almost bled out. No one could answer my wife's questions because they did not know where I was. The coup de grâce came when I was discharged at two in the morning with a prescription for painkillers that they told me to get filled at a pharmacy the next morning. As they discharged me, I asked for the best way to get back to my hotel. Although I was still heavily medicated, they told me to walk two blocks north to a major thoroughfare where I would have better luck hailing a taxi. I found a taxi, returned to the hotel, filled my prescriptions at seven in the morning, and managed to teach an all-day class that began at eight and ended at five.

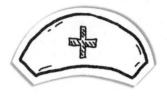

CHAPTER 4

Six Tips for Building a Partnership

The need to develop a mutually beneficial relationship with your doctor is the theme of this chapter. This can best be accomplished by taking ownership of your situation and working collaboratively with your doctor and others on the doctor's team to find a correct diagnosis and effective treatment.

Good doctors know how important it is to listen to their patients. Doctors tell their patients: "Listen to your body. If you sense that something feels wrong or a treatment is not working, tell me." Once alerted to these concerns, the doctor will know to probe more deeply—and hopefully to challenge some of his or her assumptions and consider alternative explanations for what is wrong. You need to be your own best advocate!

Doctors are more likely to succeed if you take responsibility for providing them with as much information as possible about your condition. Take time, for example, to maintain a current list of all your medications, chart your activities, and list your symptoms. Take good notes when visiting your doctor, bring previous test results with you, follow instructions carefully, and even volunteer to collect data on yourself to keep your doctor updated on your progress—or lack of it.

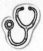

Most importantly, seek out a doctor who wants to work with you, has a reputation for listening, and can explain things to you in layman's terms. Your objective is to build a partnership with your doctor. Given the pressures he or she is under, you will learn that this is not an easy task. But the rewards can be substantial. It may turn out to be the only thing that keeps you alive!

Tap Your Network

Find a doctor who has a reputation for being a good listener and who can—and will—take the time needed to talk to you.

An essential first step in ensuring you will receive effective treatment is to find a doctor who will work with you. In talking to doctors when writing this book, all said the best way to find a good doctor is to tap your personal network of family, friends, and neighbors. Online ratings and websites can provide useful insights, but in the end, it usually comes down to two key questions: 1) How capable is the doctor (and the doctor's overall practice or institution)? and 2) How well does the doctor interact with patients? In the United States, you often need to add a third criterion: Does the doctor's practice accept your insurance?

The first question—and, to a lesser degree, the second—can often be answered by studying the doctor's website, checking biographic summaries, and perusing publications and online rating websites that rely on consumer input to rate the overall quality of medical services offered. The second question requires talking to people. When you ask someone if they can recommend a doctor, be sure to ask how well that doctor interacts with his or her patients. Treat all recommendations with skepticism until you are convinced the doctor is someone you can trust and partner with to resolve your health issues.

Once you have chosen a doctor to interview, pay attention on your first visit to how smoothly the doctor's office functions and whether you sense good chemistry among the staff. Some questions to keep in mind on a first visit include:

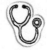

- Does the office appear to run efficiently? Are interruptions to the routine resented or accommodated?

- Were you given the opportunity to fill out all the required forms before arriving at the office?

- Is the staff friendly? Are they sensitive to your needs or special requirements?

- How good is staff morale? Are they joking with each other? How well do they support and communicate with each other?

- How good is the record keeping? Can staff quickly retrieve past tests or medical histories?

Perspective: Leveraging Your Network

When Janet was not getting better, she leveraged her network to find a better solution.

I was training to run the Boston Marathon, but it was becoming a lot harder than I imagined. Something was wrong. Sometimes when running, I would get migraine headaches and lose vision in my right eye. I started having aches and pains all over and was exhausted a lot of the time.

Visits to my medical care facility became more frequent. I was experiencing severe fatigue but no joint pain. After six months, they ran a rheumatoid arthritis (RA) panel on me, and the results suggested I had some autoimmune deficiency issues. The doctor gave me some Methotrexate pills. They really knocked me out. It was a low dose, but I stayed in bed for three days. Three months later, they prescribed a different medication, Plaquenil, but I did not improve.

When I visited the doctor's office, I noticed that no one in the reception room looked at all like me. Most of the patients had canes, and their hands were disfigured—mine were not.

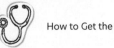

That made me think there might be a better explanation for my problem. The doctor even said I did not present like an RA patient.

After a couple years of ineffective treatment and trying several different RA medications, I was prescribed Adderall to increase my energy levels. Then they gave me Bupropion, an anti-depressant. In addition, I did a sleep study, but there were no significant findings.

Several years went by without any improvement in my condition. One day, when I was talking to a friend of mine, she said, "You don't have any eyebrows!" We are in the same running club, and we see each other most weekends. I knew she was in the medical field, but we never talked about her work. We started chatting, and I relayed that I was having problems with overall hair loss, a hoarse voice, low energy, and extremely dry skin. She said those were classic symptoms of someone with hypothyroidism. She asked me if anyone else in my family had thyroid issues, and I said, "Yes. Several of my close family members have taken thyroid medicine."

My friend encouraged me to see a doctor who specialized in treating women's hormonal imbalances. The doctor said she surmised I had an inactive thyroid after just looking at me and reading my medical history. She prescribed a natural hypothyroid medication and recommended that I slowly increase the dose. Now I self-monitor my heart rate—to calibrate how much medicine to take—and check in with my doctor every two months. I am slowly improving and feel hopeful for the first time in many years.

If you sense a lack of good chemistry or observe tension and "dropped balls" in the front office, you should start looking for another doctor. On two occasions after my major surgery, a doctor or a medical practice was recommended to me to deal with a new medical problem. When I began to use their services, I noticed some glitches in intra-office communications and, more importantly, was given advice on how to prepare for a surgical procedure that my friends said was inconsistent with practices they had followed in similar circumstances.

I learned quickly that it pays to listen to your friends. I learned how important it was to seek a second opinion, elicit recommendations from friends who had undergone the same procedure, find a good candidate, confirm that the doctor's practice could take my insurance, and set up an appointment. When I met with the new doctors, it became apparent in both cases that we had good chemistry; both also had a pleasant and engaging team supporting them. Today, I am confident both decisions to switch doctors were correct, if only because both new doctors proposed better and safer courses of treatment that ultimately proved highly successful.

List Your Symptoms

Write down your symptoms to share with your doctor, but avoid the trap of diagnosing yourself.

The primary function of a doctor is to help you get better, or, if that is not possible, help you maximize your ability to live a good life. The key to coming up with a good treatment is knowing what is causing the problem. The best way to come up with a good diagnosis is to have as complete an understanding as possible of what is different. This means your doctor needs a comprehensive list of symptoms you have experienced and the context in which they have occurred.

The preferred way to capture what is going wrong and what might have caused your problem is to write down your symptoms in advance of your visit. If you write it down and give it to your doctor, you will not have to worry that you forgot to mention an important fact. If you review the list just before your visit, you may also realize that you left something important out and can add it to the list.

Most doctors say that making such a list is one of the most important contributions patients can make toward alleviating their problem. What they find far less useful are patients who tell the doctor they know what is wrong and offer a diagnosis. Many symptoms manifest themselves for many different conditions. Once patients have convinced themselves they have illness X, they are likely to see only evidence that confirms that diagnosis. They may also ignore other symptoms that would be inconsistent with that diagnosis. Making a self-diagnosis can also be a mistake because a doctor's responsibility is to diagnose a patient's problem; your doctor may resent it when you tell him or her how to do their job.

When you see the doctor or go to the hospital, you will often be asked to rate your pain on a scale from one to ten or to point to which "smiley face" best matches how you are feeling. The idea is to give the doctor or nurse some sense of how much pain you are experiencing as an indicator of the seriousness of the problem. The practice also establishes a baseline that the doctor can refer to at a subsequent date to judge if your condition is getting better or worse and how quickly.

If a doctor asks you to rate your pain, he or she should also ask you whether you have a high or a low pain threshold. This is essential for establishing an accurate baseline. Someone with a high pain threshold, for example, may be in a lot more trouble than they think. Another good input when establishing this baseline is to describe the worst pain you have ever experienced.

Distinguishing between aches and various types of pain can also be helpful. In my experience, the pain experienced from a cut or a kidney stone attack is a lot different than the agony of a migraine or the discomfort of a swollen knee. A kidney stone attack begins as an ache as pressure builds up in the kidney but then transforms to acute pain as the stone begins to pass out of the body. Those who have suffered from a kidney stone attack know well that the ache is a trigger telling you to get to the hospital quickly, before the oncoming pain becomes unbearable.

An alternative to simply rating your pain on a scale of one to ten is to make a copy of Figure 9 and circle the word or words that best describe what you are feeling. In addition, you should tell the doctor what you do to lessen the pain and what activities seem to exacerbate it. If the doctor forgets to ask, be sure to tell him or her. The answer will make it easier for the doctor to diagnose what is actually causing the pain and how urgent it is to begin treatment.

Pain: Which word(s) describe it best?

- Unbearable
- Excruciating
- Sharp
- Shooting
- Stabbing
- Stinging
- Burning
- Throbbing
- Tender
- Slight

Aches: Do you feel it in your muscles or somewhere else?

- Numb
- Tingling
- Dull
- Gnawing
- Sore
- Tiring
- Annoying

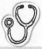

Duration: How often do you feel it?

- Constant
- Chronic
- Intermittent
- Periodic
- Episodic
- Nagging
- Occasional

Spread: Describe the phenomenon.

- Localized
- Specific
- Penetrating
- Spreading
- Radiating
- Near the surface
- Deeper inside

Figure 9. Using Words to Describe What You Are Experiencing

Again, try to avoid telling the doctor what you think is the problem; focus instead on describing how you are experiencing the discomfort. What you say will give the doctor invaluable clues into what is causing you to suffer. For example, read the following descriptions of pain and ask yourself how they differ.

- My left shoulder hurts. It's a sharp pain that's worse when I move my left arm up or to the front or back; in fact, clasping or unclasping my bra is excruciating since I have to twist my arm back. If I roll over on my left side at night, I'm awakened by a sharp, stabbing pain in my shoulder. Heat and an anti-inflammatory

(Aleve) make it feel better. I can't pinpoint a specific time that it began.

- My right leg hurts. It feels like the top of the right leg and thigh are burning and tingling; the pain feels like it's shooting down the outside of the thigh to the knee. When I'm sitting, it's more of a dull ache, but standing up or bending over makes it worse; the pain gets sharp. The only thing that makes it better is to lie down, but not on a soft mattress. It started suddenly when I turned my body to get out of my car one morning.

As you can see, the pains are distinguishable and do, indeed, have different causes. Succinctly and accurately describing your pain will help your doctor pinpoint plausible diagnoses and the most likely tests to confirm the hypothesis *(see Figure 10)*.

A good patient should do research on the Internet to learn more about his or her condition and the various illnesses associated with their symptoms. A good practice is to develop comprehensive lists of symptoms associated with what could be relevant illnesses. The key is to generate a robust list of symptoms to look for while avoiding the temptation to resolve what specifically ails you. Focus attention on the symptoms and let your doctor worry about the diagnosis and appropriate treatments.

When conducting Internet research, take care to determine the source of the information. Some websites that appear to be helpful are sponsored by the pharmaceutical industry or medical device providers and can be fraught with bias and misinformation. Figure out who sponsors or funds the website. This can provide some useful insights into whether to expect bias in how the information is presented.

When your doctor asks, "What are you feeling?" try to describe:

1. The specific location of your pain:

   - On the surface?

   - In the muscles (deeper)?

   - In the joint (even deeper)?

2. Whether it travels to other parts of the body.

3. What you are actually feeling (see *Figure 9*).

4. How it started; when you first were aware of it.

5. What makes it better.

6. What makes it worse.

7. The duration of the pain; how long have you experienced it?

8. Associated symptoms, such as weakness or numbness.

9. Whether the pain limits any of your activities.

Figure 10. Help the Doctor Find What Causes the Pain

Another Internet strategy is to do a search on your topic and include the word "complaint" or "scam" to see if any users have objected to what appears on the Internet—and whether they have good reason to do so. The best strategy is to rely only on data that is supported by multiple, independent sources over a period of several years.

Keep Detailed Notes and Bring Them to Your Appointments

Organize your own folder of previous diagnoses, test results, medical histories, prognoses, and medications that you can refer to when meeting with your doctor.

If you walk into the doctor's office with a folder full of notes under your arm, the doctor will know immediately that you are someone who wants to ensure that he or she is fully and accurately informed. Having a folder signals that you feel equally responsible for trying to diagnose your problem and want to work with your doctor to find a suitable diagnosis.

The folder should contain records of all previous tests. Before going to the doctor's office, be sure to make copies of any relevant tests that you can leave with the doctor. Your primary physician or another doctor may have already forwarded them to your doctor, but you never know. In some cases, you may have paperwork summarizing your previous diagnoses or prognoses.

In preparation for meeting your doctor, make a list of your current medications and dosages. Bring this list with you and give it to the nurse to ensure they have the most current—and most accurate—information on your medications. An example is provided in Figure 11. Be sure to include both prescription and nonprescription medications. Sometimes it is useful to provide on a separate piece of paper a list of medications you discontinued taking in recent months or during the past year.

(Patient) **Personal Medication List**				
Current as of: (Date)				
Medication	**Dose (strength, number of pills, dose)**	**Route (by mouth, inhaled, on skin)**	**Frequency (how often)**	**Purpose**
Prescription:				
Atorvastatin (Lipitor)	20 mg	By mouth	Daily in p.m.	Reduce high cholesterol
Proventil	2 puffs	Inhaled	Before running	To combat shortness of breath
Synthroid	88 mcg	By mouth	Daily in a.m.	To combat thyroid deficiency
Etc.				
Over the Counter:				
Adult Aspirin	81 mg	By mouth	Daily in a.m.	To thin blood/ heart disease
Vitamin D3	2000 IU	By mouth	Daily in a.m.	Vitamin D deficiency
Eucerin Lotion	As needed	On skin	When needed	For dry skin
Etc.				

Figure 11. Template for Making a List of Personal Medication

Another useful practice is to prepare a list of what diseases, major operations, and hospitalizations you and members of your family have experienced. You usually are asked these questions every time you visit a new doctor. It is much more efficient to maintain, print, and give your doctor a copy of your "Family History Summary" than to try to remember what to write down while sitting in the doctor's office. Creating such lists and keeping them current will take a little time upfront but will save you substantial time in the future!

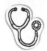

When you bring your folder, always include some sheets of blank paper so that you can write down what your doctor is telling you. Do not trust yourself to remember all the instructions you receive in the doctor's office. If a friend or member of your family accompanies you, ask him or her to take detailed notes for you. The process of writing down what you are told has two benefits:

1. It ensures you will have an accurate record of what to do.

2. It will often prompt you to ask additional questions to clarify what you need to do after you leave the doctor's office.

Perspective: Document Your Symptoms as You Build Your Folder

Sarah was falling apart, and she was told she needed surgery. With good documentation, she found a better solution.

Within four months of moving into my new condominium, I began to feel awful. My doctor attributed it to allergies that are prevalent in my part of the country. Three months later, I was suffering from migraine headaches (which I had never had before) as well as severe sinus difficulties, an inability to sleep, a horrific cough, and lethargy that left me nearly immobile. I reached a point when I could not even drive.

My internist sent me to an ENT doctor who, following X-rays, recommended me for sinus surgery. As I drove home from that appointment, I remembered a colleague who had suffered similar symptoms several years prior. He had agreed to the sinus surgery but came out of it with the same symptoms and sufferings. Sometime later, he learned he had moved into a "sick" new office building. As it turned out, he was highly allergic to dye in the carpeting.

I wondered if I might be a victim of black mold because there had been water issues in my building. Black mold can kill by spores incapacitating your immune system, shutting

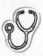

down your organs, and damaging your brain, all of which seemed to be occurring with me. I made an appointment with a different ENT to get a second opinion. I gathered all my tests, X-rays, and other papers and headed to his office, having to be driven by my daughter. I did not share with the second physician my suspicion that black mold was causing my problems. I merely told him that I was requesting his opinion regarding a recommended surgery. He looked at the tests and other documents I had in my folder. After reviewing them, he concluded, "surgery will do you no good."

Having learned his opinion, I mentioned my suspicions regarding black mold in my building. He indicated I might be right. He recommended that I move out of the building. If my suspicions were correct, he believed I would notice improvement in three-to-four weeks.

I took his advice and started to notice improvement within a month. It took a few years to get back to what I consider close to normal, but now I am a relatively healthy seventy years old, very active, and loving life.

When I visited one of my allergy and asthma doctors, I pulled out my thick yellow folder and started taking notes at the beginning of the session. In this instance, the doctor had two interns accompanying him who were similarly taking notes. Just the fact that everyone was taking notes introduced more structure into the conversation. We all knew there would be a written record of our conversation and that it was important for all of us to employ good critical thinking skills. I hope the notetaking also prompted the doctor to be more systematic in how he approached my problem and willing to suggest more creative explanations for my condition.

The process of taking detailed notes also signals to the doctor and his medical team that you intend to follow the directions and accept your responsibilities as a patient. If, on your return visit, your doctor finds out that you forgot to take a medicine as

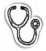

instructed or were inconsistent in following directions, he will be less incentivized to work with you to treat your condition.

When hospitals discharge patients, they review with them what medicines the patient needs to take and what procedures to follow before leaving the hospital. They also document this with written discharge instructions because they know the patient is highly unlikely to remember everything that he or she is told.

Document Your Experiences

To better focus your conversation, provide a short synopsis of what you and your doctors have already learned.

If you are starting to suspect that you are becoming a member of the "5 percent club" who cannot get a diagnosis or effective treatment for your condition, then chances are high you will be visiting more doctors in the future. A good technique for making those visits more efficient (and hopefully more productive!) is to write a short history summarizing all that you have endured. Begin with a list of your symptoms and then describe which doctors in which specialties you have seen, what tests you have taken with what results, and what treatments have been tried with what, if any, success.

The synopsis should not be too short in that it leaves out critical information, nor too long in that it contains unnecessary detail. A good target is to keep the draft to three-to-five pages, single-spaced. The synopsis should be tightly organized and flow easily from one paragraph to another. You will know you have achieved this goal if you can give it to someone to read and their eyes never wander off the paper until they have read the entire thing. If the reader stops to ask you questions, you should find a way to answer the question succinctly in a revised version. If the reader loses concentration while reading your story, you need to improve the flow and probably delete some extraneous verbiage. Another check on your writing skills is to read only the first sentence of

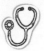

every paragraph and ask yourself if those sentences accurately and succinctly tell your story.

In some circumstances, consider adding a few documents as an appendix. For example, you could provide the results of a recent test or a list of all the doctors you have engaged and their specialties. In some cases, you might want to provide a chronology or timeline or even a list of diagnoses that have been considered and abandoned for various reasons.

I did not recognize the benefit of crafting your own personal narrative until almost the end of my odyssey. Fortunately, my family doctor had proposed that I submit my case to the NIH Undiagnosed Diseases Program. The application process required me to summarize my case history, which covered most of the information fields mentioned above. I had placed this three-page report in my thick yellow folder and had it with me when I drove to the emergency room.

When the ER doctor told me for the second time that I should go home, my three-page "story" quickly became my last line of defense. I pulled it out of my yellow folder and asked him to read it. If it had been a long treatise or a sheaf of unorganized documents, I doubt he would have paid it any attention. When he saw that it was only a three-page document, he must have calculated he could afford the few minutes to read it. It took him only three minutes to read the entire thing. Thankfully, it was sufficiently well-organized and compelling for him to keep reading to the end. The paper had its intended impact, making the doctor more willing to admit me for further testing.

Offer to Collect Data on Yourself

Ask your doctor what information you can collect at home that would help him or her come up with the correct diagnosis.

Doctors need data to help them make a diagnosis. The primary sources of data are test results and what their patients tell them. As discussed previously in this chapter, patients should bring a list of symptoms to give to their doctor at their first meeting as well as a list of current medications and family medical history. In most cases, more data will be needed before the doctor can make a diagnosis.

Sometimes, additional information is obtained through further testing, but often people can generate useful data on their own. For example, a dietician will ask you to keep a record of everything you eat for a given week, or a physical trainer will ask you to record how many hours of exercise you get every day. You may also decide to buy a blood pressure meter at the local pharmacy and maintain a list of your readings on an Excel spreadsheet to show (or email to) your doctor. It helps to take a reading using your meter right before and after your appointment with your doctor. Then you can compare readings to determine if either is not calibrated correctly.

Perspective: It Pays to Track What You Eat!

Nothing the doctors ordered fixed Helene's eye problem until a stranger told her what not to eat.

For many years, I would get inexplicable swelling and "weeping" in my eye along with inflammation and redness. I went to an ophthalmologist who said it was blepharitis, a condition that can only be treated with expensive steroid creams that cost more than a hundred dollars for a small tube. A second doctor prescribed the same steroid cream but called the problem ocular rosacea—a hereditary condition for which there is no cure. A third doctor said my eye looked so bad that he suspected it was infected. He prescribed an antibiotic cream to take along with the expensive cream. But the problem did not get better.

The epiphany came in a women's restroom on a military base. As I was carefully applying the eye cream, a stranger came up behind me and asked, "Do you eat eggs? I recognize that eye cream. It is really expensive and does not do a bit of good. I spent hundreds of dollars on that cream before I realized I needed to stop eating eggs. You have an egg allergy, trust me. Stop eating anything made with eggs. You won't regret it."

At that moment, I realized I had been eating scrambled eggs almost every day. Traveling constantly, I had little choice but to eat mostly "buffet-style" breakfasts at motels and military bases. I wanted to eat "healthy," so I would pile up my plate with scrambled eggs instead of those sugary Danishes and nitrite-laden bacon. As soon as I stopped eating eggs, the "ocular rosacea" and the so-called eye "infection" completely disappeared. To this day, I know when something has egg in it because my eyes get red, and I look like I have been crying.

Another advantage of collecting data on yourself is that the process serves as a constant reminder of the need to eat healthy, exercise regularly, develop a personal network, and get enough sleep. In this day and age, there are far too many temptations, and you can easily succumb to a poor diet of processed and genetically modified foods, chemicals, and other preservatives— none of which are good for your body. If you monitor your food intake and track how much time you devote to exercise and other healthy activities, you will bring more happiness and less stress into your life.

Perspective: Connecting with Your Doctor

The doctors said further treatment would not save my sister's life, but Joan refused to accept that decision. How could I convince the doctor to keep trying?

We were in the hospital, grasping at straws, in total disbelief. The test results showed that my forty-six-year-old sister's breast cancer had metastasized to her brain and spine.

We debated the depressingly narrow range of options left for her care. One doctor told us that no matter what we did, all efforts were likely to prove futile. Another presented a very limited set of options, and we decided to continue treatment. My sister was not going to take "no" for an answer. She had so much to live for. She said, "If I am going down, it won't be without a fight!" She said she would take the last swing and wanted us to advocate on her behalf for all that could be done—even after she was unable to make that decision for herself. We promised her that we would do exactly that for her at each turn.

After all treatments were complete, the doctors told us there was nothing left to do. This message confused us because she had improved a great deal. How could they be terminating treatment now? During the final visit from her radiation oncologist, I noticed he was wearing a crucifix around his neck. I felt a strong personal connection to him as I am Catholic. I recognized the crucifix as an opportunity to connect and appeal to him on new grounds. I asked if we could speak privately in the hallway.

In the hallway, I asked him if he was Catholic. He was initially taken aback by my question, but kindly answered, "Yes." I told him that I was struggling not only over the potential loss of my sister, but as an individual marked with the sign of Catholic faith. As a Catholic, I was taught to value life as a precious gift from God. I believed we have a duty to protect life until we die, even though this duty is not absolute. I asked of him, as a Catholic, to please consider a range of additional options appropriate for my sister's care if there was any hope of improvement in her condition.

From that moment on, the doctor seemed to personally take on the mantle of making my sister improve. He spent more time at her bedside with our family and checked in on her more frequently.

I don't know if the exact course of treatment was different based on our conversation or whether he would have recommended additional radiation despite my personal plea. What I do know is that the conversation forged a personal connection between the doctor and our family and, most importantly, my sister. It gave her the hope she needed

*to fight for as long as she did. He provided her with the gift
of giving her that last swing. And as far as she knew, she
delivered cancer the final blow.*

Create Incentives

*Find ways to incentivize your doctors and their staff to pay more
attention to you.*

Most doctors see tens of patients every day. Your challenge is
to find ways to make yourself and your case stand out among
the crowd. If it makes sense for your child to bring an apple to
school for the teacher, why not do the same for your doctor? One
doctor told me it really got his attention when a patient sent him
a Christmas card—and he never forgot the person who texted him
with a festive Happy Birthday greeting. While such acts sound
trivial, we all are human. Often it is the little things in life that
you remember.

Another strategy is to find common ground with your doctor. Are
you an alumnus of the same college or university? Do you share
the same religion, go to the same church? Do you support the
same charities? Do you live in the same neighborhood? Do your
children go to the same school? How well does your doctor know
the person who recommended him or her to you?

Early in my saga, I knew that two of my doctors were runners
like me. I looked for opportunities to share stories about running
with them. I also knew they were busy people and surmised they
probably did much of their running on the weekend. Since my
problem was connected to running, I thought it would make sense
to offer to run with them one weekend so they could observe my
frustrations firsthand. They took the suggestion seriously, but in
the end, we failed to make it happen.

Another strategy I tried on two occasions was to propose that
my doctor and I write a joint, publishable article on my condition.
I was an accomplished author and methodologist, and they

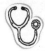

were experts in their field. Both of us would benefit greatly from adding another published article to our résumés. I calculated that they would not only be more incentivized to focus attention on my problem but would be increasingly motivated to come up with a solution we could document in our jointly authored article. Moreover, I would have no problem giving them first mention on the byline! Both doctors found the idea intriguing, but no publishable article was produced. I attribute this in part to the vagaries of the publishing world. Another reason could have been their inability to figure out what was wrong with me. A good story should always have a satisfying ending.

The key is to find a way to establish a personal connection with your doctor so that you stand out a little from the crowd. Ideally, whatever strategy you employ would not only advantage your doctor but create shared benefits or opportunities for both of you.

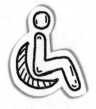

CHAPTER 5

An Unexpected Outcome

Early in the morning on March 11, 2014, the nurses prepared me for a routine surgical procedure. The doctor inserted a small camera into a large blood vessel in my groin and routed it up a major artery to check out the condition of my heart and surrounding arteries. I was told doctors were reluctant to prescribe this procedure, called a catherization, because of the potential for complications with an invasive procedure. The good news for me was that I could watch the catherization on a monitor. Unfortunately, I lacked the expertise to interpret what the screen was displaying.

A Surprise Diagnosis

When the procedure was completed, the cardiologist came to speak with my wife and me. He showed us a diagram of the heart and all the main arteries. In my case, the heart muscle itself was normal, but both major arteries—the right coronary artery (RCA) and the left main coronary artery (LMCA)—were seriously calcified. The RCA had a 70 to 80 percent blockage. The main coronary artery (MCA) had a 40 to 50 percent blockage as it entered the heart and another 80 percent blockage just below that.

The MCA has two branches. My cardiologist pointed out that the left anterior descending branch, also known as "the widow maker," was 60 to 70 percent blocked. The right branch was also 70 percent blocked. More critically, he believed a new clot had recently created a 90 percent blockage in the widow maker just above the 70 percent blockage. We speculated that this blockage occurred while I was in Barcelona. It was that blockage that had made it difficult for me walk to the State Department without losing my breath (see Figure 12).

The doctor said that surgery was urgently needed and told me I needed to undergo a quadruple heart bypass operation immediately. He recommended that I remain in the hospital. They scheduled the surgery for early the next morning.

A More Surprising Response

My reaction took the doctor by surprise. It can be summed up in one word: "Yippee!" I had been struggling for years and was increasingly frustrated that no one could tell me what was wrong with me. Now, the answer was crystal clear. My heart was strong, and the hospital had a great reputation. Moreover, the cardiology unit was one of the best in the country. Nevertheless, the doctor told me that no one in the hospital could remember anyone celebrating being told they needed quadruple bypass surgery.

As I was being wheeled to my room in the cardiac ICU after the surgery, the cardiologist approached my wife and told her he wanted to apologize to her and to me on behalf of the profession of cardiology. He said it was apparent that I had been misdiagnosed from the start, and my doctors had done me a disservice. She graciously accepted his apology.

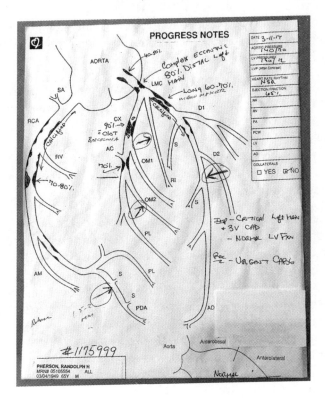

Figure 12. Extent of Arterial Blockage

The cardiologist explained that one of the reasons they misdiagnosed me was that I had a "balanced ischemia" that often is not caught on nuclear treadmill tests. Most treadmill tests are designed to look for contrast, and all my arteries were fairly equally damaged. As a result, the tests did not show enough contrast to be sufficiently alarming. My condition was a rare occurrence as the hospital had encountered only a few patients with similar histories in the past ten years.

In hindsight, my case was a classic example of the power of the cognitive bias called Anchoring. Once a cardiology team had determined that I did not have a heart problem, this conclusion was accepted as gospel and the search began to find alternative explanations. Every subsequent doctor focused solely on whether

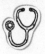

my problem could be ascribed to something emanating from his or her specialty, be it asthma, some other lung condition, an allergy, my throat, or another cause entirely.

My wife and I decided not to alert anyone to my situation until I came out of surgery. I was surprised that the doctors and nurses allowed me to continue to run my businesses over my iPhone literally until I was wheeled into surgery. They then took the phone from me, put a sticker on it, and placed it under my bed. It was there for me when I came out of surgery, but I was in no condition to start using it!

The surgery lasted four hours. I came out of anesthesia by late afternoon, but still was fairly groggy. I was determined to communicate many new ideas, however. A tube had been placed down my throat, which made it impossible to talk, so I drove my family crazy trying to write words on a sheet of paper or spell them out with my finger. I thought I was surprisingly articulate given my condition. My wife was not as convinced. She had the foresight to save the paper I wrote on (see Figure 13). Clearly, she had the more accurate perception of my state of mind.

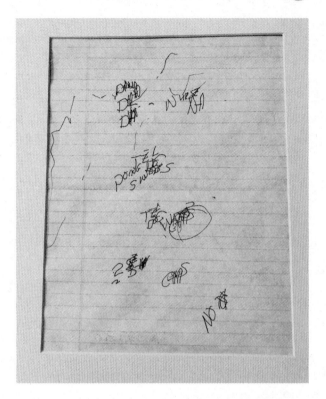

Figure 13. Trying to Communicate After Heart Surgery

A Quick Recovery

I recovered quickly. As a good analyst, one of the first things I did was to count how many wires and tubes connected me to the instruments and outlets on the wall behind me. I stopped counting at fifty-eight. My goal was to reduce that number to a handful. I managed a short walk around the cardiac ICU ward the day after the surgery. On the second and third days, I did several laps. I was released to go home three days after the operation. Once home, I managed to stop taking opioid painkillers six days after leaving the hospital. I stopped taking Tylenol (500 mg) within twenty days.

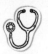

On March 18, just as I was going off my painkillers, my primary care doctor received a letter from the NIH Undiagnosed Diseases Program. The letter was their response to my request that they accept me into the program. The director of the program informed me that:

> After careful consideration, it was decided by the medical review board that we would not be able to invite your patient to participate in our program. The program's goals are to provide answers to patients with mysterious conditions that have long eluded diagnosis and to advance medical knowledge about rare and common diseases. The medical team bases its judgment on whether or not there is a reasonable chance to achieve these goals.

After the first week, I began to walk slowly on a treadmill at my gym, increasing my time a little bit each day. When I reported for physical therapy, the physical trainers at the hospital determined that I had already surpassed the targets they would have set for me and signed a release. I was happy they waived my need to return for any workouts because it was an hour drive from my home and my gym was only five minutes away!

A major milestone was passed when my doctor signed a form giving my extremely capable personal trainer permission to take over my rehabilitation. We resumed our twice-weekly workout sessions, but at a much less aggressive pace. She had a specialty in rehabilitation exercise, and she guided me through a program that allowed me to progress rapidly and, more importantly, avoid any relapses.

Ten days after my surgery, I asked my doctors what I could do to further accelerate my recovery. They said the most important thing was to walk long distances on a flat surface. Unfortunately, our house is in a hilly neighborhood, and we have no sidewalks— so I came up with a better solution.

Twelve days after my surgery and after receiving grudging permission from my doctors, I flew to Toronto, Ontario, to present papers on three different panels at the International Studies Association (ISA) conference. My justification for the trip was that it enabled me to take advantage of twenty-six kilometers of flat, underground arcades—a perfect venue for extensive walking.

Initially, I doubted I would be able to stand to present my papers. At the last moment, I decided I could stand if I used the podium to maintain my balance. On the third day of the conference, I hosted a reception put on by my company and was happy to sit down once it concluded.

I could accomplish these tasks because I was accompanied by two dear colleagues who had volunteered to push my wheelchair through the airport, carry my books when walking down the hallways at the conference, and accompany me to various events. It was a pleasant surprise to see how quickly one could pass through the various airport security lines when in a wheelchair! At the ISA conference the following year, many attendees who had interacted with me in Toronto were amazed to learn that I had undergone heart surgery only two weeks before the previous conference.

Within a month of the surgery, I felt almost fully recovered, but I recognized the need not to push myself too far. My heart was as strong as ever, I had four new arteries, and I had developed a supporting network of minor capillaries to move blood through my system. My chest was healing nicely, but my legs were a little numb where three arteries had been "borrowed" to replace the bad ones next to my heart.

I received permission to start walking with my running club and even to jog downhill on smooth pavement. A couple weeks later, I started running a little on flat pavement. To be honest, I was in no hurry to start running up hills! My doctor's main concern was that I not fall and crack my chest open. He convinced me that a chest bone repair operation was to be avoided at all costs. I knew that within a few more months, I would once again be able to go on

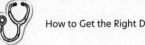

a five- or ten-mile run and feel the endorphins kick in after the three-mile mark.

Today, if someone asked me to distill all that I learned over the course of my five-year odyssey into five lessons learned, they would be the following:

1. Advocate for your own health care; treat your doctor as your partner in the adventure.

2. Press your doctor to offer a diagnosis and, preferably, to offer more than one!

3. Focus on how best to describe your symptoms; let your doctor do the diagnosing.

4. Seek a second opinion if you have any concerns about proposed treatments.

5. Find creative ways to spur your doctor—and the doctor's team—to distinguish you from the crowd.

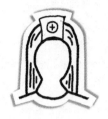

Engaging Your Doctor

If you want to live a long and healthy life, the most important thing you can do is to advocate for your own health care. A list of the most important actions you can take is provided at the end of the previous chapter.

The first step in this process is to take responsibility for helping your doctor diagnose your problem. The medical industry is highly incentivized to press doctors to order tests and emphasize treatments. This strategy is highly cost efficient and, I suspect, may ensure that as many as 95 percent of the general population is appropriately treated.

The problem lies with how the remaining 5 percent are treated. If incentives are lacking to focus on finding a correct diagnosis, then most of us who belong to the "5 percent club" will die without getting a proper diagnosis. And when most of us die, few will ask if good medicine could have prevented the deaths. A cause of death will be cited, and the family will be too overcome with grief to ask if the medical profession abdicated its primary function—to make a proper diagnosis.

The best way out of this dilemma is to find doctors who will remain curious about your condition and are willing to challenge their assumptions and explore unlikely possibilities. Once you have found a good doctor, advocate for your own health care. Offer to partner with your doctor to find the best diagnosis.

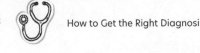

Another strategy is to convince a nurse to advocate for you. He or she has spent more time at your bedside than the doctor and is in a good position to evaluate your needs.

Dr. Atul Gawande, author of *Being Mortal*, takes it to a higher level. He contends that doctors should not just strive to provide a correct diagnosis, but should ask their patients what their goals are.[23] Patients should discuss what risks they are willing to take and what they most want out of life. A technique he uses is to ask patients, "Once we deal with your condition, how would you describe your best possible day?" The answers to this question should determine what prognosis to pursue in optimizing quality of life for the patient.

Propagating the Message

Another strategy to consider is to incorporate courses or segments of courses in medical degree programs to teach the critical thinking skills discussed in this book. A strawman agenda for such a course is provided in *Figure 14*.

The course begins with an exploration of the cognitive biases and intuitive traps doctors and nurses are most likely to fall victim to. This discussion is followed by a series of exercises giving the students practice in using five core structured techniques: Key Assumptions Check, Multiple Hypothesis Generation, Analysis of Competing Hypotheses, Indicators, and Deception Detection. Students then pair up to conduct role-playing exercises on how to communicate more effectively with patients. The workshop concludes with a capstone exercise focusing attention on the five habits doctors and nurses should instill into their daily routines and thought processes.

23   Atul Gawande, "Being Mortal's Villages: The Value of Community and Choice as We Grow Older," live-streamed conversation, Beacon Hill Villages Event, Temple Rodef Shalom, McLean, VA, September 25, 2017.

Day One

- Introduction
- Analytic Traps and Mental Mindsets
  - Exercise: Identifying Key Cognitive Biases and Intuitive Traps
- Techniques for Overcoming Mindsets
  - Exercises: Key Assumptions and Generating Multiple Hypotheses
- Analysis of Competing Hypotheses or Differential Diagnosis
  - Exercise: Developing Checklists of Disconfirming Indicators

Day Two

- Detecting Deception
  - Role-Playing Exercise for Anticipating Deception
- Improving Collaboration and Teamwork
  - Role-Playing Exercise for Communicating with Your Patient
- The Five Habits of an Effective Practitioner
  - Capstone Exercises: Practicing What You Have Learned
- Wrap-Up: Key Takeaways

Figure 14. Intelligence Tradecraft for Medicine: Strawman Course Agenda

Appendix A: Multiple Hypothesis Generation

Multiple Hypothesis Generation is a structured way to generate a comprehensive set of mutually exclusive hypotheses for explaining a particular problem, condition, or behavior.

Multiple Hypothesis Generation is part of any rigorous analytic process because it helps people avoid common pitfalls such as coming to premature closure or being overly influenced by first impressions. It helps you think broadly and creatively about a range of possibilities. The goal is to develop a mutually exclusive and comprehensively exhaustive list of hypotheses that can be scrutinized and tested against existing symptoms, test results, other information, and any new data that may become available in the future.

The Multiple Hypothesis Generation technique is a useful tool for broadening the spectrum of plausible hypotheses. It is particularly helpful when there is a prevailing lead hypothesis and little thought has been given to alternative possibilities. It is also helpful when there are several members of the medical team, none of who can agree on what should be the lead diagnosis.

The Process

1. Succinctly define the medical case, illness, problem, activity, or behavior that is under examination.

2. Establish the lead diagnosis or "hypothesis" for explaining this problem, activity, or behavior.

   - The lead hypothesis could be the one you were given, the most obvious explanation, or the conventional wisdom.

3. Critically examine the lead hypothesis by identifying and

listing its key components.

- Use the journalist's classic list of Who, What, When, Where, Why, and How to evaluate all critical dimensions of the lead hypothesis.
- Some of these questions may not be appropriate for the particular problem or behavior you are examining.

4. Generate plausible alternative explanations for each key component.

- Once this process is complete, you should have lists of alternative explanations for several components of the lead hypothesis.
- Strive to keep the alternative explanations on each list mutually exclusive.

5. Identify all the possible permutations that can be generated using these lists.

6. Discard any permutation that simply makes no sense.

7. Evaluate the credibility of the remaining hypotheses by challenging the key assumptions of each component.

- Some of these assumptions may be testable themselves.
- Assign a "credibility score" for each hypothesis, e.g., using a 1 to 5 point scale.

8. Re-sort the remaining hypotheses, listing them from most to least credible.

9. Select from the top of the list those alternative hypotheses most deserving of attention (and inclusion in an Analysis of Competing Hypotheses matrix, if appropriate).

Hypothesis Generation Example

1.   **Issue Definition:** Why are Navajos living in the Four Corners region of the United States dying suddenly?

2.   **Lead Hypothesis:** Healthy young Navajos living in the Four Corners region are dying from exposure to a virulent form of a common flu virus.

3.   **Key Component Identification**

     a) Who was dying?

     b) What caused their death?

     c) How did they become ill?

4.   **Generate Alternative Explanations for Each Component**

     - **Who was dying?**

       a) Only members of the Navajo nation.

       b) People living in the Four Corners region, including Navajos.

     - **What caused them to become ill?**

       a) A virulent form of the common flu.

       b) Unknown disease (natural pathogen).

       c) Leakage of a chemical toxin processed at nearby Fort Wingate.

     - **How did they become ill?**

       a) Act of nature.

       b) Intentional act of man.

       c) Accidental exposure.

5.   **List All Possible Permutations**

     A list of all possible permutations is provided in *Figure 15*.

6. **Discard Permutations that Make No Sense**

    For example:

    - Only Navajos are dying from accidental exposure to a virulent form of the common flu.

    - Someone is using a virulent form of the common flu to kill people.

    - Only Navajos are dying from accidental exposure to a chemical toxin.

7. **Rate the credibility of the remaining hypotheses and**

8. **List them in rough order of plausibility.**

    For example:

    a) People are dying from a virulent form of the common flu.

    b) Someone is using an unknown pathogen to kill Navajos.

    c) Someone is using a chemical toxin to kill Navajos.

    d) Only Navajos are dying from a naturally occurring chemical toxin.

9. **Select from the List Those Hypotheses Most Deserving of Attention (and for Possible Inclusion in the Analysis of Competing Analysis Matrix, if Appropriate)**

    a) People are dying from a virulent form of the common flu.

    b) People are dying from a naturally occurring, new, unknown pathogen.

    c) Someone is using a new, unknown pathogen to kill people.

    d) Someone is using a new, unknown pathogen to kill Navajos.

e) People are dying from accidental exposure to a new, unknown natural pathogen.

f) People are dying from accidental exposure to a chemical toxin.

Who	What	Why	Permutations	Credibility Score
Only Navajos	Virulent Form of the Common Flu	Act of Nature	Only Navajos are dying of a virulent form of the common flu.	discard
		Intentional Act of Man	Someone is using a virulent form of the common flu to kill Navajos.	discard
		Accidental Exposure	Only Navajos are dying from accidental exposure to a virulent form of the common flu.	discard
	Unknown Disease (Natural Pathogen)	Act of Nature	Only Navajos are dying from a new, unknown natural pathogen.	
		Intentional Act of Man	Someone is using a new, unknown natural pathogen to kill Navajos.	
		Accidental Exposure	Only Navajos are dying from accidental exposure to a new, unknown natural pathogen.	discard
	Chemical Toxin	Act of Nature	Only Navajos are dying from a naturally occurring chemical toxin.	
		Intentional Act of Man	Someone is using a chemical toxin to kill Navajos.	
		Accidental Exposure	Only Navajos are dying from accidental exposure to a chemical toxin.	discard

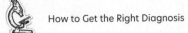

Anyone	Virulent Form of the Common Flu	Act of Nature	People are dying of a virulent form of the common flu.	
		Intentional Act of Man	Someone is using a virulent form of the common flu to kill people.	discard
		Accidental Exposure	People are dying from accidental exposure to a virulent form of the common flu.	discard
	Unknown Disease (Natural Pathogen)	Act of Nature	People are dying from a naturally occurring unknown new pathogen.	
		Intentional Act of Man	Someone is using a new, unknown pathogen to kill people.	
		Accidental Exposure	People are dying from accidental exposure a new, unknown natural pathogen.	
	Chemical Toxin	Act of Nature	People are dying from exposure to a naturally occurring chemical toxin.	
		Intentional Act of Man	Someone is using a chemical toxin to kill people.	
		Accidental Exposure	People are dying from accidental exposure to a chemical toxin.	

Figure 15. Example of Multiple Hypothesis Generation: Death in the Southwest Case Study

Credibility Score

Discard	Not logical
1	Low Credibility
3	Medium Credibility
5	High Credibility

Appendix B: Analysis of Competing Hypotheses

ACH is a tool to aid judgment on issues requiring careful weighing of alternative explanations, hypotheses, or diagnoses. ACH involves the identification of a complete set of alternative explanations (presented as hypotheses or diagnoses), the systematic evaluation of each, and the selection of the explanation that fits best by focusing on information that tends to disconfirm rather than confirm each of the explanations.

Doctors face the perennial challenge of working with incomplete, ambiguous, anomalous, and sometimes deceptive information. In addition, strict time constraints and the need to "make a call" often conspire with natural human cognitive biases and intuitive pitfalls to produce inaccurate diagnoses. ACH improves the doctor's chances of overcoming these challenges by requiring her or him to identify and refute all but one credible alternative explanation based on known symptoms, laboratory tests, assumptions, knowledge gaps, and other pertinent information.

The Process

Step 1. Create a matrix.

Step 2. Identify all the possible diagnoses or hypotheses and list them at the top of each column in the matrix. Be sure that they are mutually exclusive and comprehensively exhaustive.

Step 3. List all significant pieces of relevant information (symptoms, test results, validated assumptions) in the rows going down the left side of the matrix. (Include any conspicuous absence of evidence.)

Step 4. Indicate in each cell whether the relevant information is highly consistent with, consistent with, inconsistent with, highly inconsistent with, or is not applicable to each diagnosis.

Consider information as highly inconsistent if the item makes a compelling case that the diagnosis must be incorrect. Similarly, list information as highly consistent if a compelling case can be made using this information to show the diagnosis is correct.

Step 5. Discount all diagnoses where the listed inconsistent information makes a persuasive case for dismissing the hypothesis.

Step 6. Determine how sensitive the lead diagnosis(es) is to a few critical items of relevant information. Consider the consequences for the analysis if that finding were wrong, misleading, or subject to a different interpretation.

Step 7. Identify key facts or future actions the team should explore to distinguish between the lead diagnois(es) or increase confidence that the chosen diagnosis is correct.

Figure 16 shows how ACH was used to determine why relatively healthy people of all ages in the Four Corners region of the United States were dying suddenly. Substantial inconsistent information was found to negate the lead hypothesis that people were dying from a highly virulent form of a common flu virus. Significant inconsistent information was also found to cause one to question two other hypotheses: 1) Navajos were the targets of a hate crime, and 2) the deaths were related to exposure to a toxic substance processed at Fort Wingate. The remaining hypothesis, that a new, little know pathogen, a hantavirus, was responsible for the sudden outbreak of unexpected deaths, was confirmed by the Centers for Disease Control.

	H:4 Navajos Succumb to New Pathogen	H:2 Exposure to Toxic Substance	H:3 Navajos Target of Hate Crime	H:1 Virulent Common Flu Virus
Weighted Inconsistency Score ⇨	-1.0	-3.0	-5.0	-10.0
Enter Evidence				
E6 Tests for comon flu and bacterial agents are negative	C	I	I	II
E11 Victims had abdominal/back pain with low blood platelet counts	CC	I	I	I
E7 Some people treated with antibiotics recovered	I	N	I	I
E16 No reporting of anti-Navajo rhetoric on internet	NA	N	II	NA
E10 Surveys show not all had visited the same places	N	I	N	I
E12 Many symptoms consistent with presence of toxic substance	N	CC	C	I
E4 Young, healthy adults dying	C	C	C	I
E3 Almost all victims are Navajos	C	C	CC	I
E2 Medical personnel are not becoming infected	C	C	C	I
E1 Victims have flu-like symptoms with quick progression to respiratory distress and death	C	C	C	I
E15 Recent wet winters and 10-fold increase in rodent population	C	NA	NA	N
E14 Powerful disease linked to wet winters and increased rodents	C	NA	NA	N
E13 Many died suddenly of similar powerful disease in 1918 & 1933	C	NA	NA	N
E9 Most patients live in Four Corners area	C	C	C	C
E8 Ft. Wingate munitions storage and demo facility nearby	N	CC	C	NA
E5 High mortality rate	C	C	C	C

Source: Sarah M. Beebe and Randolph H. Pherson

Figure 16. Example of the ACH Method: Death in the Southwest Case Study

Appendix C:
Indicators Generation

Indicators are a pre-established set of observable phenomena (or symptoms) that are monitored and assessed to confirm or disconfirm the viability of a diagnosis.

Preparation of a detailed list of indicators or symptoms to track provides a useful learning experience for all participants. It facilitates the exchange of knowledge among those on the medical team and can spur a decision to order new tests or conduct additional research. The identification and monitoring of confirming and disconfirming indicators can spur early warning of untoward developments or unanticipated changes in the condition of the patient. The human mind tends to see what it expects to see and to overlook the unexpected. Indicators take on meaning only in the context of a specific diagnosis with which they have been identified.

The Process

Step 1: Working alone, or preferably in a small group, brainstorm a list of indicators that would confirm the validity of the diagnosis(es). Also, create a list of indicators that would demonstrate that the favored diagnosis is incorrect *(see Figure 17)*.

Step 2: Review and refine both sets of indicators for each diagnosis(es), discarding in each set any that are duplicative and combining those that are similar.

Step 3: Examine each indicator to determine if it meets the following five criteria. Discard those that are found wanting:

- **Observable and Collectible.** There must be some reasonable expectation that, if present, the indicator will be observed and reported to the medical team.

If an indicator is used to track whether change has occurred over time, it must be collectible over time.

- **Valid.** An indicator must be clearly relevant to the stated diagnosis and accurately measure the problem, illness, or phenomenon at issue.

- **Reliable.** Data collection must be consistent when comparable methods are used. Those observing and collecting data must observe the same things. Reliability requires precise definition of the indicators.

- **Stable.** An indicator must be useful over time to allow comparisons and to track events. Ideally, the indicator should be observable in the near future so that the doctor has time to react accordingly should contrary indicators prove the diagnosis to be incorrect.

- **Unique**. An indicator should measure only one thing, and in combination with the others, should point only to the selected diagnosis and never to any alternative diagnoses previously considered.

Lead Diagnosis:

Criteria:

- a. Observable and Collectible
- b. Valid
- c. Reliable
- d. Stable
- e. Unique

Candidate Confirming Indicator	A	B	C	D	E
Candidate Disconfirming Indicator	A	B	C	D	E
1.					
2.					
3.					
4.					
5.					

Figure 17. Indicators Generation Worksheet

Appendix D: Key Assumptions Check

A Key Assumptions Check is a group exercise to list and challenge the working assumptions that underlie a key judgment or diagnosis.

Assumptions are unavoidable and necessary.

- It is reasonable to take certain things for granted.
- It is sometimes necessary to make assumptions until confirmation comes.
- Estimations and complex problems often require simplifying assumptions to make them manageable.

The quality of an assumption, however, can range from poor to good. Much depends on the basis of the assumption. Over the years, facilitators have observed that approximately one in four key assumptions usually collapses on careful examination.

The Process

Step 1. Assemble a small group. Gather a small group of people who are familiar with the case, along with one or two "outsiders" who can come to the table with an independent perspective. An "outsider" is someone who does not know much or anything about the patient or the case but understands what the group is trying to accomplish. Ideally, the group would include a few doctors and nurses, the patient, one or two family members, and an intern or health professional not familiar with the case.

Step 2. Define the key objective. If necessary, provide the participants with a short summary of the case one or two days before the session. Ask them to identify two or three assumptions that are likely to underlie the analysis. When the group is

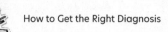
assembled, briefly review the case and answer any questions. Develop a consensus on the objectives of the session.

Step 3. Ensure agreement on the definition of an assumption. An assumption must be true for another condition or development to be valid; it can also be a fact or statement that people will take for granted. The latter are often generated by cultural bias or reflect an entrenched mindset.

Step 4. List your key assumptions. On a whiteboard or an easel, list all the assumptions identified by the participants. Resist the temptation to critique the assumptions as you list them (see Figure 18).

Key Assumption	Rationale	Rating: Solid (S), Caveated (C), or Unsupported (U)
1.		
2.		
3.		
4.		
5.		
6.		
7.		

Figure 18. Key Assumptions Check Worksheet

Solid: An assumption that is basically supported.

Caveated: An assumption that is correct with some explicit caveats.

Unsupported: An assumption that is unsupported or questionable.

Step 5. Evaluate the assumptions. After developing a complete list, go back and critically examine each assumption. Encourage the participants to ask themselves the following questions.

You may want to display these questions on another easel or a whiteboard or provide it as a handout.

- How much confidence do I have that this assumption is valid?

- Why do I have this degree of confidence?

- Under what circumstances might this assumption prove untrue?

- Could it have been true in the past, but is no longer true today?

- If it turns out to be invalid, how much impact would this have on the diagnosis?

Step 6. Categorize the assumptions. Place each assumption in one of three categories:

1. Basically **solid** or well-supported (i.e., self-evident or common sense).

2. Correct, with some **caveats** (i.e., based on history, doctrine, or "normal" behavior).

3. **Unsupported** or questionable (i.e., entirely hypothetical or even far-fetched—I could wake up tomorrow to find out it was wrong and understand why).

Figure 19 provides an example of this process as used in the Death in Southwest Case Study.

Step 7. Identify Key Uncertainties. Some Unsupported Assumptions may turn out to be Key Uncertainties. These uncertainties should be noted for follow-up testing or research.

Step 8. Organize the list of assumptions. Group the assumptions into three categories—Solid, Caveated, and Unsupported. Prioritize the assumptions in each group.

Step 9. Consider next steps. Ask the group if it would be appropriate to take the list of Key Uncertainties and possibly

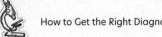

some of the caveated assumptions and generate a list of things to do to resolve the uncertainty. What additional tests should be ordered, what questions should be asked, and what new research is needed?

Step 10. Generate a final product. After the session, circulate a list of prioritized assumptions and any future actions that the group is spurred to take as a result of the brainstorming session.

Key Assumption	Rationale	Solid	Caveated	Unsupported
1. Cause of death is a highly potent flu virus	Symptoms similar to flu but would have to be a form unique to the area		√	
2. Disease could spread quickly	A genuine concern, but no evidence of spread beyond Four Corners			√
3. Disease has unusually high mortality rate	Most of those who contract disease die within a few days	√		
4. The rapid deaths suggest a terrorist act	There is no evidence that terrorists were targeting the Four Corners area			√
5. Illness can be treated with antibiotics	Some treated recovered, but no proof this was because of the antibiotics		√	
6. Most of the victims are Navajos	The preponderance of those dying are members of the Navajo nation	√		
7. Navajos are being targeted	There is no evidence that someone is intentionally targeting Navajos			√
8. Exposure to a toxic substance caused the deaths	Many of the symptoms correlate with exposure to a toxic substance		√	
9. Dead Navajos were victims of a hate crime	There is no evidence to support this			√
10. The disease is not contagious	To date, no medical personnel have fallen ill from the disease		√	
11. Rodents are known carriers of disease	Rodents are known carriers of many diseases with similar symptoms	√		
12. Rodent population grew tenfold 1992-93	A fact documented by ecological researchers	√		

Figure 19. Example of a Key Assumptions Check: Death in the Southwest Case Study

Appendix E:
Premortem Analysis

Premortem Analysis is conducted prior to finalizing an analysis or diagnosis by a doctor or, preferably, a medical team, to brainstorm how the chosen diagnosis could be spectacularly wrong.

The goal of Premortem Analysis is to challenge—actively and explicitly—an established mental model or analytic consensus in order to broaden the range of possible explanations or diagnoses that are being seriously considered. This process helps reduce the risk of analytic failure by identifying and analyzing the features of a potential failure before it occurs.

The Process

Step 1. Gather in a room all those who are involved in the process of making a diagnosis or have a vested interest in the diagnosis being correct.

Step 2. Tell the group to imagine that some time has passed since the diagnosis was made and the patient has since died, or his or her condition has deteriorated in a totally unexpected and dramatic way. No one now challenges the conclusion that the diagnosis was wrong—it was a spectacular mistake!

Step 3. Engage the team in using a brainstorming technique—such as Cluster Brainstorming or Circleboarding™—to explore plausible explanations for this unexpected outcome. Try to identify all the possible ways the analysis could be wrong. Encourage everyone to come up with ideas. Sometimes a silent brainstorming technique is preferable, such as passing out notecards and asking each participant to write down one or two ideas. Then, collect all the cards and write the ideas on a

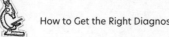

whiteboard or an easel. Challenge the group to see who can come up with the best idea of how a misdiagnosis came about.

Step 4. Look for patterns or groups of ideas and revisit your conclusions and evidence to see if you have overlooked, misinterpreted, or ignored key information.

Step 5. Decide if any alternative diagnoses merit attention, and whether any new tests should be administered or additional research conducted.

If sufficient time is not available to work through this entire process, a fallback strategy would be to add the following question to a list the doctor uses before he or she comes up with a diagnosis: *Six months has gone by and the patient has died. What would explain how this happened?*

Appendix F: Structured Self-Critique

A Structured Self-Critique is a systematic procedure that a small team or group can use to identify weaknesses in its own analysis.

When conducting a Structured Self-Critique, all members of the medical team don a hypothetical "black hat" and become critics of their own analysis. From this perspective, the medical team responds to a list of questions about sources of uncertainty, the analytic processes used to arrive at the conclusion(s), assumptions made, the diagnosticity of evidence, information gaps, changes in the broad context in which events happened, alternative decision models, potential deception, and cultural expertise.

When questions are asked about the same topic but from this critical perspective, team members often give a different answer than they gave before. For example, if a team member is asked if he or she supports the team's conclusions, the answer will usually be "yes." However, if all team members are asked to look for weaknesses in the team argument, the same team member may give a quite different response.

This shift in the frame of reference is intended to change the team dynamics. By embracing a critical perspective as a group, the team is more likely to discover flaws in the analysis. Team members who may have previously suppressed questions or doubts because they lacked confidence are now empowered by the technique to express divergent thoughts. If this change in perspective is handled well, each team member will know that they have added value to the exercise by being critical of, instead of supporting, the previous judgment.

Structured Self-Critique can help both patients and the medical team mitigate mistakes they might have made at several steps in the diagnostic process. The process of questioning the key building blocks of the analysis can uncover faulty assumptions, differences in evaluating evidence, information gaps, and other weak or incorrect elements. Deliberately "poking holes" at an argument can be challenging and difficult for authors or team members, particularly if they have worked an account or on a patient for a long time. Forcing the members of a unit, team, or group to do so can reveal unconscious bias, such as the examples listed below (see Figures 20 and 21).

Mirror Imaging	Assuming that others will act the same as we would, given similar circumstances.
Groupthink	Choosing the option that the majority of the group agrees with or ignoring conflicts within the group due to a desire for consensus.
Fundamental Attribution Error	Overrating the role of internal determinants of behavior (personality, attitudes, beliefs) and underestimating the importance of external or situational factors (constraints, forces, incentives).

Figure 20. Sample Cognitive Biases to Consider

Projecting Past Experiences	Assuming the same dynamic is in play when something seems to accord with past experiences.
Imposing Lessons Learned	Selecting a hypothesis only because it avoids a previous error or replicates a past success.
Relying on First Impressions	Giving too much weight to first impressions or initial data, especially if they attract our attention and seem important at the time.

Figure 21. Sample Intuitive Traps to Consider

A Structured Self-Critique exercise is helpful when a Premortem Analysis raises unresolved questions about the viability of the original diagnosis. The medical team may also find a Structured Self-Critique a useful double check when dealing with a particularly difficult case. It can help resolve issues when members of the team have conflicting opinions.

The Process

Step 1. Remind all participants that they are now wearing "black hats" and their job is to be critics—not advocates—of the team's analytic conclusions. Their job is to find weaknesses in the analysis. Can the diagnosis stand up to brutal scrutiny? Ask the following questions in conducting the critique:

- *Sources of Uncertainty:* Should we expect to find: a) a single, obviously correct answer; b) a most likely answer, together with one or more alternatives that should also be considered; or c) a number of possible explanations that merit attention?

- *Analytic Process:* In the initial analysis, did the team do the following: Did it identify potential alternative diagnoses and seek more information on these diagnoses? Did it seek a broad range of diverse opinions by including others not familiar with the case in the deliberations? If not, this increases the odds of the team having a faulty or incomplete analysis. Either consider doing some of these things now or lower the team's level of confidence in its judgment.

- *Critical Assumptions:* How recent and well-documented is the evidence that supports the assumptions made in this case? Brainstorm circumstances that could cause each of these assumptions to be wrong and assess the impact on the team's analytic judgment if an assumption is wrong. Would the reversal of any of these assumptions support any alternative diagnosis?

- *Diagnostic Evidence:* What lead diagnosis did we identify, and what are the most diagnostic items of evidence that have enabled the team to reject the alternative diagnoses? For each item, brainstorm one or more reasonable alternative interpretations of the evidence that could make it consistent with an alternative diagnosis.

- *Information Gaps:* Are there gaps in the available information, or is some of the information so dated that it may no longer be valid? Is the absence of information readily explainable? How should it affect the team's confidence in its conclusions?

- *Missing Evidence:* Is there any evidence that one would expect to see in the interviews of the patient and the tests performed if the diagnosis is correct, but which is *not* there?

- *Anomalous Evidence:* Is there any anomalous item of evidence that would have been important if it had been believed or could have been related to diagnosis, but was rejected as unimportant or not significant? If so, try to imagine how this item might be a key clue to an emerging alternative diagnosis.

- *Changes in the Broad Environment:* Might any social, technical, economic, environmental, or political changes play a role in why this particular diagnosis was chosen?

- *Alternative Decision Models:* Were any judgments based on a rational actor assumption? If so, consider the potential applicability of other decision models, specifically that the action was the result of standard organizational processes or the whim of a close-minded or overly stressed doctor. If time to do a more thorough analysis is lacking, consider the implications of that for confidence in the team's judgment.

- *Cultural Expertise:* Is the team or one of its members unduly influenced by cultural factors or ignorant of cultural norms that may be associated with the problem?

- *Deception:* Would the patient or anyone on the team have motive, opportunity, or means to engage in deception to influence what diagnosis was made? Does the patient have a history of engaging in deception or lying about his or her past behavior?

Step 2. Based on the answers to the themes of inquiry outlined above, list the potential deficiencies in the evidence and logic that support the diagnosis in order of their potential impact on the correctness of the diagnosis.

Step 3. Discuss what the group could have done to avoid any of the potential flaws in thinking discovered during the Structured Self-Critique exercise.

This technique will not be effective unless participants understand that everyone's appropriate role is to find fault with or pick apart the analysis, assumptions, and evaluation of evidence. Even if they know the intent of the exercise, some participants will have difficulty divorcing themselves from the original findings and conclusions.

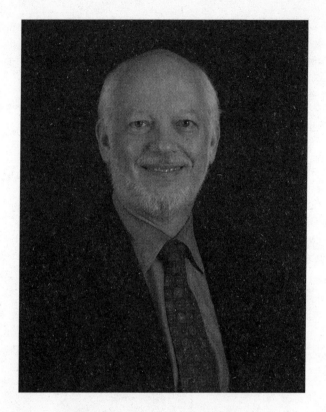

About the Author

For over a decade, Randolph H. Pherson has been developing and teaching Structured Analytic Techniques and critical thinking and writing skills to analysts throughout the intelligence, homeland security, and defense communities as well as in the private sector and overseas. Since retiring from the CIA in 2000, he has authored, coauthored, and edited ten books, most recently publishing the *Analyst's Guide to Indicators* and the *Handbook of Analytic Tools & Techniques, 5th edition*. He is best known for coauthoring *Structured Analytic Techniques for Intelligence Analysis* with Richards J. Heuer Jr. and *Critical Thinking for Strategic Intelligence* with his wife, Katherine Hibbs

Pherson. He has an AB from Dartmouth College and an MA in International Relations from Yale University.

As Chief Executive Officer of Globalytica, LLC, Mr. Pherson has developed and taught courses in over two dozen countries, supporting major financial institutions, global retailers, and security firms. In recent years, he has facilitated over two dozen Foresight Analysis workshops for foreign governments, international foundations, and multinational corporations. His company provides training in both the classroom and online, including an Intelligence Analyst Professional program that is certified by the International Association for Intelligence Education. As President of Pherson Associates, Mr. Pherson has been actively engaged in teaching and mentoring analysts across the US Intelligence Community as well as consulting with senior intelligence officials on how to develop robust analytic cultures. Mr. Pherson is a Founding Director of the Forum Foundation for Analytic Excellence, a nonprofit established in 2011 to promote the effective use of critical thinking skills and Structured Analytic Techniques by teaching, certifying, and applying these skills to a broad range of enduring and emerging issues.

Mr. Pherson worked for twenty-eight years in the US intelligence Community, last serving as National Intelligence Officer for Latin America. His mission was to provide the most objective and insightful analysis as possible to senior US policymakers, based on the available reporting and solid logic. While at the CIA, he served on the Inspector General's staff, as Chief of the Director's Strategic Planning and Management Staff, and as Executive Assistant to the Executive Director of the Agency. He is the proud recipient of the Distinguished Intelligence Medal for his service as NIO for Latin America, the Distinguished Career Intelligence Medal, and several other meritorious citations.

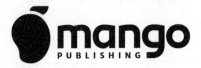

Mango Publishing, established in 2014, publishes an eclectic list of books by diverse authors—both new and established voices—on topics ranging from business, personal growth, women's empowerment, LGBTQ studies, health, and spirituality to history, popular culture, time management, decluttering, lifestyle, mental wellness, aging, and sustainable living. We were recently named 2019's #1 fastest growing independent publisher by *Publishers Weekly*. Our success is driven by our main goal, which is to publish high quality books that will entertain readers as well as make a positive difference in their lives.

Our readers are our most important resource; we value your input, suggestions, and ideas. We'd love to hear from you—after all, we are publishing books for you!

Please stay in touch with us and follow us at:

Facebook: Mango Publishing

Twitter: @MangoPublishing

Instagram: @MangoPublishing

LinkedIn: Mango Publishing

Pinterest: Mango Publishing

Sign up for our newsletter at www.mangopublishinggroup.com and receive a free book!

Join us on Mango's journey to reinvent publishing, one book at a time.